Posture and Movement of the Child With Cerebral Palsy

Marcia Stamer, PT

Illustrations by Delilah R. Cohn, Kathleen Jung, and Diane L. Nelson

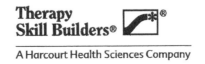

Therapy Skill Builders®

A Harcourt Health Sciences Company

Library of Congress Cataloging-in-Publication Data

Stamer, Marcia Hornbrook.

Posture and movement of the child with cerebral palsy:
a guide for physical, occupational, and speech therapists /
Marcia Stamer; illustrations by Delilah R. Cohn, Kathy Jung,
and Diane L. Nelson.

    p.   cm.

Includes bibliographical references and index.

ISBN 0-7616-4900-X (alk. paper)

1. Cerebral palsied children—Rehabilitation. 2. Movement
disorders in children. 3. Posture disorders in children.
4. Cerebral palsy—Exercise therapy. I. Title.

[DNLM: 1. Cerebral Palsy—rehabilitation—Child. 2. Movement—
Child. 3. Occupational Therapy—Child. 4. Physical Therapy—
Child. 5. Posture—Child. 6. Speech Therapy—Child. WS 342
S783p 2000]

RJ496.C4 S83 2000

618.92'836—dc21   00-012229

 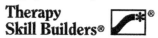

Dedication

Especially for Annie Watwood

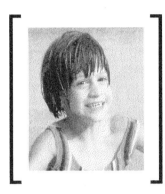

January 11, 1989 – June 23, 1997

Though your time on earth was short and your challenges great, you communicated your uniqueness in a moment to all who had the pleasure of knowing you. I will always remember how hard you worked, how easily you smiled, and how clever you were when your plans were different from mine! You will always be greatly loved and cherished.

This book is dedicated to all the children I have ever had the pleasure of working with in therapy and to their families. It is with these children and their families in mind that I undertake this project, in the hope that we all will gain a better understanding of the needs of children with cerebral palsy. And though I believe it imperative that we understand those needs, I hope that we always keep the perspective that the children we work with are still children, with all the joy and challenges any child brings to this world.

> "If you start off saying a child is special because she suffers from a handicap, that is a disservice, because you are robbing her of what she might become on her own. We too often disguise the truth by employing that word. . . . We are all made different. We make ourselves special."

> —Frank Deford, father and author
> *Alex: The Life of a Child*

Acknowledgments

There are many people I have learned from over the years whose knowledge of the needs and treatment of children with cerebral palsy are now so much a part of mine that I know this work is not solely my own. Foremost is *Judi Bierman, PT,* who taught me so much, both in the classroom and in the clinic. Many other Neuro-Developmental Treatment instructors, peers, and students in my continuing education classes have contributed more than they will ever know.

I would like to thank *Barbara Cupps, PT,* and *Lois Bly, MA, PT,* for encouraging me to write this book after they saw a long series of outlines on the subject of development in children with cerebral palsy that I use in my continuing education courses.

I want to thank *Linda Hillman, PT; Monica Wojcik, MA, CCC-SP;* and *J. Lyndelle Owens, CCC-SP;* for reviewing, correcting, and suggesting positive changes when my manuscript was in progress.

I also would like to thank *Allison Whiteside, PT,* who thoroughly read and edited the first draft of this book. Her suggestions were always valuable, and she deserves credit for making me think even harder and for suggesting positive changes to the wording and meaning of the text.

About the Author

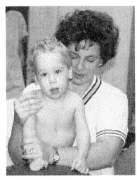

Marcia Stamer, PT, received her Bachelor of Science in Physical Therapy from Ohio State University in 1980. Her intensive continuing education background includes training in the Neuro-Developmental Treatment (NDT) approach, the Advanced Baby Course, and the Maitland Approach to Spinal Mobilization. She is a certified Coordinator/Instructor of the NDTA, Inc./Bobath Eight Week Pediatric Course in the Treatment of Children with Cerebral Palsy. Marcia is a member of the APTA and Pediatric Section, the AACPDM, and the NDTA. Her teaching experience includes many continuing education workshops on various pediatric topics, such as manual therapy, dorsal rhizotomy, gait, children with severe physical involvement, and various types and ages of children with cerebral palsy using the NDT approach.

Ms. Stamer has practiced in Canton, Ohio, and Augusta, Georgia. She has worked with children in multidisciplinary center-based settings, school settings, outpatient hospital care, and in ICF/MRs.

Ms. Stamer also is the author of *Functional Documentation: A Process for the Physical Therapist* and contributed four articles regarding children with hypotonic, hypertonic, athetoid, and ataxic cerebral palsy to *Parent Articles About NDT.*

Ms. Stamer and her family currently live in Nashville, Tennessee. She teaches continuing education courses related to children with cerebral palsy, consults with area therapists in treatment settings, and is an adjunct clinical instructor in the School of Physical Therapy at Belmont University in Nashville, Tennessee.

About the Artists

Delilah R. Cohn, M.F.A., Certified Medical Illustrator, received her B.S. in Medical Illustration from the University of Illinois Medical Center in Chicago in 1971 and an M.F.A. in illustration from Syracuse University in 1984. She is board certified, past Secretary of the Board of Governors for the Association of Medical Illustrators (AMI), and recipient of the AMI Outstanding Service Award in 1998. She was employed in the medical illustration department of State University of New York, Upstate Medical Center in Syracuse until 1979 and subsequently founded The Medical Illustration Studio. Ms. Cohn has created illustrations for many medical textbooks, journals and presentations, for a permanent exhibition on human embryology for the Cumberland Science Museum in Nashville, TN, and for medical-legal cases.

Kathleen Jung, M.S., Certified Medical Illustrator, earned her B.S. in Medical Art from the University of Illinois at the Medical Center in Chicago in 1971 and her M.S. in Health Science Education from Case Western Reserve University in Cleveland, OH, in 1980. Ms. Jung is a member of the Guild of Natural Science Illustrators and the Association of Medical Illustrators. She is board certified and currently serves on the AMI Board of Governors. She has been a medical illustrator at the Loyola University Medical Center in Chicago and the Cleveland Clinic Foundation in Cleveland. Currently she runs a freelance business illustrating medical textbooks and professional journals and is an Associate Professor of Medical Illustration at the Cleveland Institute of Art and an adjunct Associate Professor in the Department of Anatomy of Case Western Reserve University.

Diane L. Nelson, M.H.P.E., Certified Medical Illustrator, has been a professional medical illustrator for 30 years and her work has been published in professional journals, medical textbooks, and anatomical charts. Ms. Nelson's professional affiliations include the Association of Medical Illustrators, for which she served as President and Chairman of its Board of Governors. She has also served on the National Certification Board of Medical Illustration and is currently a Clinical Assistant Professor at the University of Illinois at Chicago, Department of Biomedical Visualization. Among awards and distinctions Ms. Nelson has received are Awards of Excellence from the Association of Medical Illustrators and the Annual Rx Club Show, Certificate of Excellence from the American Institute of Graphic Arts, and Best of Show Award in Illustration from the Bio-communication Chicago Forum.

Contents

Contents

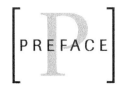

PREFACE

Although children with cerebral palsy have been treated in physical, occupational, and speech therapies for decades, detailed, comprehensive descriptions of their development, learning, impairments, functional limitations, and disabilities are rarely found in the literature. Even more rare are clinically applicable treatment ideas for therapists.

My understanding of children with cerebral palsy is based on clinical experience, discussion with and observation of peers treating children with cerebral palsy, and critical reading of the literature. Hopefully, the descriptions in this book can be used to generate research ideas that will enrich our understanding of the needs of children with cerebral palsy.

My hope is that clinicians who read this book will feel that they have more detailed information, more options for treatment, and a system with which to evaluate the children they care so much about. I hope, too, that researchers will gain ideas for specific studies that will test the truth of the descriptions in this book. Although writing and revising a book is a tremendous task, it would bring me great pleasure to revise these descriptions again based on solid research findings. Better understanding is the basis of better treatment.

Although children with cerebral palsy are unique individuals with their own strengths and needs, this book divides and classifies cerebral palsy into categories based on distinct pathophysiologies. In reality, most children with cerebral palsy do not fit into neat classifications as far as their strengths, impairments, functional limitations, and disabilities are concerned. This book is organized by these classifications only to assist you in identifying the groups of impairments, functional limitations, and disabilities that often are seen together. While this can help you organize your observations, analysis, and treatment planning, it only begins the process of carefully thinking and planning for each individual child.

Each child with cerebral palsy is different from the next. The child has a unique family, personality, and strengths. Find out about those first. The child will never fit this book. We are the best we can be as therapists when we start by valuing and caring about each child as a unique person. Then you can use this book to help yourself learn more about the posture and movement dysfunction of the child you treat. Believe your observations and the child's family's observations and goals, then work to learn why you see what you see and what you will do about it.

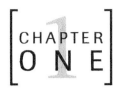

CHAPTER ONE

Introduction

History and Terminology

Cerebral palsy (CP) is defined as a group of non-progressive, but often changing, motor impairments due to lesions of the central nervous system (CNS) in the early stages of development (Kuban & Leviton, 1994). Although the lesion itself is non-progressive, the resulting impairments, disabilities, and handicaps can be progressive. One reason for this is that a lesion has an impact on a body, and hence a CNS, that is still growing and maturing. In addition, the impairments, disabilities, and handicaps interact over time, producing further changes and impairments.

Cerebral palsy was first identified in the literature by Dr. William Little, who described it in detail in a paper presented to the London Obstetrical Society in 1861 (Schleichkorn, 1987). The disability was first called Little's disease because of his extensive descriptions and early attempts to determine the causes of what he called spastic infantile paralysis. He attributed CP mainly to perinatal events and abnormal birth processes. Sigmund Freud also described cerebral palsy in the 1890s (Newton, 1995) and did some of his early work in this field. He challenged Little's concept that cerebral palsy usually was caused during the birth process. Freud felt that it was not always possible to determine when in the development of the fetus and neonate the insult(s) took place. He suggested that perhaps problems in fetal development were sometimes the cause of an abnormal birth process.

Early in this century, CP was treated using primarily an orthopedic approach. Surgery that was used for children with polio often was used for children with cerebral palsy. According to Dr. Winthrop Phelps, an orthopedist of the period who devoted extensive time to children with CP, such surgery had disastrous results. He believed in bracing and in organizing teams of professionals to treat children with cerebral palsy (American Academy for Cerebral Palsy and Developmental Medicine [AACPDM], 1996).

In the 1940s, new approaches for treatment emerged in the world of therapy. These approaches looked more holistically at the many impairments caused by the CNS lesion and expanded treatment beyond what physicians were already doing. New treatment ideas by the Bobaths, Margaret Rood, and others also came into being (Levitt, 1995). These approaches attempted to understand the problems in sensory and motor control and the role that development played in attaining skills, as well as the secondary orthopedic impairments caused by CP. These pioneers established clinical and theoretical treatment and management strategies for therapists. Their work was revolutionary—they firmly believed that with therapy people with CNS lesions could alter their anticipated prognosis. The beliefs of these practitioners had such a profound impact on the world of therapy that it often is taken for granted today that our treatment is beneficial. (We are well advised to look critically at the results of everything that we do, however!)

Historical Perspectives on the NDT Approach to Treatment of Children With Cerebral Palsy

Because there is such widespread misunderstanding of the NDT approach, even in the literature (Olney & Wright, 1994; Ostrosky, 1990; Sahrmann, 1983; Van Sant, 1983), it is wise to look historically at its development. Much of the criticism is based on the belief that practitioners who use the approach today still adhere to the theoretical assumptions made in the 1940s and 1950s about motor control. Whether or not therapists embrace or reject the concepts of the NDT approach to treatment of children with cerebral palsy, it is important that they completely understand the development of and changes in the approach.

Berta and Karel Bobath were a physician-therapist husband and wife team who worked in London (Schleichkorn, 1992). Beginning in the 1940s, they developed ideas for treatment that differed from orthopedic management only, and began publishing and teaching these ideas, eventually opening their own clinic. Berta Bobath was a physiotherapist who saw that children with cerebral palsy had more than simply muscle weakness and contracture. She observed abnormal development of motor milestones as well as deviant postures and movements, and she began to try to figure out how and why this was happening. She also saw abnormal tonus and believed that her treatment affected this tonus. Her husband, Dr. Karel Bobath, searched the literature to find explanations for these observations. He studied the neurophysiology of the day, including the work of Jackson, Magnus, and Sherrington (Bobath & Bobath, 1972). These scientists described the reflex as the basic unit of motor control and saw the CNS as hierarchically organized. They used this model of motor control to perform experiments and to explain motor behavior.

The Bobaths believed that spasticity, or hypertonus, was a release phenomenon, as explained by the neurophysiologists they studied, but they viewed this hypertonus as a release of inhibition of whole patterns of movements or postures, not just a release of inhibition of individual muscle activity. They explained changes in a child's postural activity, changes in the resistance to movement, and greater ease in movement as changes in postural tone.

The Bobaths became widely known for this new concept that the tone and the outcome of movement in children with cerebral palsy could be changed for the better. They also wrote a descriptive text on the different types of CP (Bobath & Bobath, 1975). The Bobaths' work offered hope that the outcome of children developing with cerebral palsy was not immutable, that there was the possibility of changing the way they moved. They never claimed that they could cure or eliminate the disability, however (Scrutton, 1991). Later in their careers, the Bobaths recognized that what they ultimately wished to change were functional skills.

As noted above, the Bobaths based their explanations of clinical procedures and outcomes on the neurophysiology of the day—that what they were changing was muscle tone, and that they were influencing primitive and mature reflexes. Dr. Bobath also discussed the influence of normal reciprocal inhibition—the normal relationship of muscle activity around a joint as a body segment grades movement. He and Mrs. Bobath addressed the lack of variety of movement synergies that children with cerebral palsy develop. As newer explanations of motor control emerged the original neurophysiological explanations on which the Bobaths based treatment became outdated (Shumway-Cook & Woollacott, 1995). However, because their clinical observations were innovative and astute, the newer theories of motor control, motor learning, and motor development often fit in quite well with their treatment plans.

It is likely that many aspects of reflexive and voluntary control are involved in the *tone* Mrs. Bobath discussed. Her technique of facilitation and inhibition through handling the child provides organized, graded sensory input (proprioceptive, tactile, visual, auditory, vestibular). Therefore, she may have influenced postural control and coordination through an ability to bias muscle groups to increase or decrease their firing. She helped children who needed more cocontraction to hold postures to perform more effectively. She also helped children who sustained holding postures too much to move with more graded control. She helped children initiate movement more effectively. She paid careful attention to the alignment of the body while asking a child to hold a posture or move a body segment, which probably biased the child to initiate movement more efficiently and often with more effective muscle synergies. All this she called "changing tone" because the neurophysiology of the day did not yet have more precise words.

Therapists who use the NDT approach today find that many of the explanations for the selection of treatment techniques can be very different from those originally offered by Dr. Bobath's theories, in part because we have revised our understanding of how the impairments of cerebral palsy affect a child's function. There are often new or revised neurophysiological theories that explain clinical findings in different therapeutic approaches drastic alteration of clinical applications. Therefore, it is not surprising that the NDT approach to treatment has been, and continues to be, revised.

Many of Mrs. Bobath's teachings still apply today—careful observation and evaluation; use of handling to facilitate desired movement and to obtain correct alignment for initiation of muscle activity, with gradual withdrawal of this handling as the child takes over; treatment in functional situations; and involvement of the family in treatment. The Bobaths' treatment strategy of guiding children to move in more efficient and functional ways fits quite well with today's theories of motor control and motor learning.

The Bobaths called their approach Neuro-Developmental Treatment, and it is still known by that name today. Those familiar with today's NDT often find it an excellent approach for sound clinical observation and reasoning. Its attention to individualized goals and treatment strategies is both challenging and rewarding, and its attention to function as outcome is sound rationale for treatment.

Current Neuro-Developmental Approach to Treatment of Children With Cerebral Palsy

The Bobaths' treatment philosophy is an excellent problem-solving format for understanding the needs of children with cerebral palsy. The current neuro-developmental treatment (NDT) approach has been revised and expanded to reflect more current theories of motor control (Styer-Acevedo, 1994). Currently the NDT approach encompasses several important concepts.

1. The child is evaluated as a unique individual who lives in a particular family with unique needs. The child's current and future living situations are considered when planning treatment goals. The goal of treatment is an increase in functional skills.

2. The therapist uses the knowledge of normal development to understand the many and varied ways that children develop skills. This knowledge is applied to children with cerebral palsy to understand why the child cannot perform

certain skills. Normal development no longer is used as a measure of success of treatment or even as the desired outcome of treatment. Children with CP will not follow the normal developmental milestones.

Normal developmental scales can be used to determine whether a problem exists. These scales never were intended for use as a measure of treatment success. Therapists must be wary of any research that claims that therapy is ineffective because children with CP fail to make gains on scales of normal development.

3. Because we are treating a movement disorder, treatment is an active process. Movement skills require the integration of many body systems. Therefore, treatment identifies the problems the child has with movement and how those problems affect function. The systems that affect movement must be treated simultaneously because each system's problems usually impact one or more of the other body systems. These systems include the neuromuscular system, sensory and perceptual systems, musculoskeletal system, and respiratory system. Treatment involves the decreasing input of the therapist, both physical and verbal, so the child will take over movement and learn how to initiate movement.

4. Treatment is a team approach. No one professional or family member is trained or licensed to manage all of the possible impairments, functional limitations, and disabilities associated with children with CP. Effective management involves communication among all concerned with the child.

Research and Terminology

Today there is a growing need and desire to understand more fully the long-term outcomes of any type of medical, educational, and social treatment of people with disabilities. The health care system in the United States is rapidly changing and will continue to undergo many revisions. Those who treat people with disabilities are aware of the tremendous task of making a difference in their clients' function through treatment. American health care and culture look for fast results and quick cures. Clinicians who work with people with disabilities know that there are no fast results and for many disabilities, there are no cures. Treatment, however, can make a difference in the lives of many people who have disabilities.

Several national and international organizations are working to set up systems of common understanding, terminology, and measurement of outcomes of treatment of people with disabilities. The purpose is to have a more unified language in describing disabilities and a method of research into the outcomes of treatment. The World Health Organization (WHO) and the National Center for Medical Rehabilitation Research (NCMRR) are two of these organizations that are working to define terms used to describe the problems encountered by people with disabilities.

These terms are now common in peer-reviewed literature. They also fit in well with organized clinical documentation (Stamer, 1995) and the NDT approach when describing children with cerebral palsy. This text will use these terms, in order to be current with and conform to rehabilitation research and classification. The following definitions are from the National Institutes of Health's Research Plan for the NCMRR (U.S. Dept. of Health and Human Services, 1993):

Pathophysiology: Interruption of, or interference with, normal developmental processes or structures.

Impairment: A loss or abnormality at the organ or organ system level of the body.

Functional Limitation: Restriction or lack of ability to perform an action in the manner of, or within the range consistent with, the purpose of an organ or organ system.

Disability: Limitation in performing tasks, activities, and roles to levels expected within physical and social contexts.

Societal Limitation: Restrictions attributable to social policy or barriers (structural or attitudinal) that limit fulfillment of roles or deny access to services and opportunities associated with full participation in society.

Other terms defined by the NCMRR:

Function: The performance of an action for which a person or thing is especially fitted or used.

Habilitation: An initial learning of skills that enables an individual to function in society.

Rehabilitation: Restoring or bringing to a condition of health or useful and constructive activity, usually involving learning new ways to do functions that were lost.

The NCMRR (U.S. Department of Health and Human Services, 1993) goes on to give examples of some of the terms as they apply to cerebral palsy:

Pathophysiology: Abnormal development of or perinatal injury to the central nervous system.

Impairment: Excess muscle contraction, excess reflex activity, poor control of balance and posture.

Functional Limitation: Slow and inefficient movements. Difficulties with activities of daily living such as eating, dressing, and hygiene.

Disability: Lacking independence in mobility. Not independent with family or peers. Requires assistance for school and recreational activities.

Societal Limitation: Examples include lack of full integration in school activities, lack of health insurer coverage for payment of powered wheelchair.

This text will use these terms as it describes in detail the development and characteristics of the different types of cerebral palsy. By using these terms we have a common language with others in the rehabilitation field worldwide.

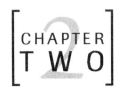

CHAPTER
T **W** O

Cerebral Palsy—The Clinical Picture

Do Children With Cerebral Palsy Develop in a Predictable Way?

There is a wealth of literature describing *selected* impairments, functional limitations, disabilities, and societal limitations placed on children with cerebral palsy. There is research targeted at understanding and/or treating certain impairments. It often is implied that if we treat the impairments successfully, a change in function can result. Other researchers are not so certain of this relationship.

Despite the abundance of literature, there is still very little in the way of basic descriptions of children with CP (Olney & Wright, 1994). Many clinicians with experience treating people with cerebral palsy have a good sense of their impairments, limitations, etc., have little written information to turn to for further reference. Many clinicians also feel that because of their impairments children with CP often develop motor skills in predictable ways. This is the theory that is taught in the NDT courses given throughout this country and around the world. Mrs. Bobath wrote about her impressions of development in children with CP (Bobath, 1985; Bobath & Bobath, 1975), and while her work provides one of the few descriptions of children with various classifications of cerebral palsy, it may need to be revised based on current understanding of motor control. However, the child who survives a premature birth or other traumatic birth today and develops with CP is likely to be very different than a child who was able to survive 10 years ago. Therefore, descriptions of children with the diagnosis of cerebral palsy must be constantly revised.

Treating Children With Cerebral Palsy

As a therapist working with children with CP, your job is to identify and treat their movement problems in order to help them achieve functions that are not likely to develop if left untreated. You need three basic skills when trying to help a child with cerebral palsy learn new and challenging functions. First, understand the impairments, functional limitations, and possible disabilities that the child has. Second, predict outcomes of such children with or without treatment. Third, develop basic treatment strategies to address those problems.

Most children with CP have a complex array of impairments and functional limitations. Their problems are complex enough that therapists with a great deal of expertise often find that their perceptions change as they constantly assess the child they are treating. Although this book is divided neatly into chapters that delineate the problems of children with hypotonia, hypertonia (quadriplegia, diplegia, hemiplegia), athetosis, and ataxia, the reality is that most children with CP cannot be placed into neat categories. Many children are hypertonic with athetosis and maybe some ataxia, or athetoid with hemiplegia or hypertonic limbs with a very hypotonic trunk. Over the 20 years that I have been treating children with cerebral palsy, the *typical* picture of hypotonia, hypertonia, athetosis, and ataxia has changed. This may be due to the change in the type of child who survives a traumatic infancy. These children often are born earlier, creating the possibility of different types of damage to organ systems because of immaturity. They also may suffer insults to their central nervous system and other systems on multiple occasions—in utero, at birth, and in the first months of life. There also are full-term children who are born with damage to various organ system which may have once been fatal, but for which the technology now exists that enables these children to survive.

Separating types of CP into chapters, however, gives the reader a way to sort out the impairments, postures and movements, and functional limitations seen in children with one classification of cerebral palsy. This helps therapists understand the likely results of certain pathophysiologies (diagnoses). At the least, it offers therapists a framework in which to begin to look at children with cerebral palsy.

Using the NCMRR Model of Disablement
Pathophysiology

There are many approaches to understanding the damage that the lesions of cerebral palsy can cause children. In the past, the NDT approach and other neurological approaches used a hierarchical theory of central nervous system organization and attributed the damage and resultant movement disorder to "released" lower-level CNS control (Gordon, 1987). These released lower-level centers were believed to result directly in the impairments seen in children with cerebral palsy. Examples of this are spasticity, tremors, involuntary movements, hypotonia (decreased excitability of the stretch reflex), and abnormal synergies of movement. These examples of release of more primitive and automatic movements are termed positive signs of CNS dysfunction. In other words, these signs are abnormal reflexive tone states or abnormal movements not seen in people with intact central nervous system functioning.

Negative signs of CNS damage are losses or deficits thought to be the results of direct damage to motor control areas of the CNS (Sahrmann & Norton, 1977), which causes a loss of motor control function. In other words, the child has lost something that he should have. Examples are loss of cocontraction or loss of reciprocal inhibition, delayed termination of motor unit activity, prolonged sustaining of firing of muscle activity (loss of the ability to terminate this activity), and restricted range of movement. Many researchers find a more direct correlation of these negative signs of CNS dysfunction to the child's skill level than positive signs to the child's skill level (Carmick, 1995b; Davis & Kelso, 1982; Eliasson, Gordon, & Forssberg, 1991; Sahrmann & Norton, 1977; Sugden & Utley, 1995).

Assumptions about why a child moves the way she does when she has cerebral palsy must take into account these negative signs. Treatment approaches and techniques must shift from treating or seeing only the positive signs as the causes of dysfunction to evaluating and treating the negative signs. The NDT approach to treatment has changed its focus to looking at these negative signs in a disablement model structure.

For example, Davis and Kelso (1982) question the relationship of hypotonia to movement disorder in children with Down syndrome. Hypotonia is a positive sign. In their experiments, Davis and Kelso showed that the differences in motor control between young men with Down syndrome and those without any CNS deficits were due to losses (negative signs)—that is, loss of precision of movement due to underdamping and loss of the ability to regulate neuromuscular stiffness with movement. Shumway-Cook and Woollacott (1985) also found the problems of movement in children with Down syndrome to be those of negative signs rather than the positive sign of hypotonia. In fact, they found the motor neuron pool excitability of children with Down syndrome to be comparable to that of children with normal development. They also found that children with Down syndrome showed delayed initiation of postural sway (loss of the speed of initiation of movement) during standing platform studies.

The emphasis of this manual is to describe the possible losses (negative signs) seen clinically in children with cerebral palsy. Because these often are based on observations rather than research, I can only hypothesize what these losses are in the different types of CP and try to correlate them to possible functional skill losses.

Impairments

Impairments that are likely to be present in each classification of CP are divided according to each system affected by the pathology of the lesion. This is in accordance with NCMRR's definition of impairment as "a loss or abnormality at the organ or organ system level of the body."

Research has shown that the lesions that cause cerebral palsy most often cause damage to more than one system, resulting in impairments that influence movement control (Borzyskowski, 1989; Castle, Reyman, & Schneider, 1979; Fuji et al., 1987; Harada et al., 1993; Laplaza & Root, 1994). Primary impairments are those that are immediately and directly a result of the lesion. Secondary impairments develop in systems or organs over time because of the effects of one or more primary impairments, and may become just as debilitating as those primary impairments.

Anyone who treats children with cerebral palsy notices that many things get worse, not better. What often gets worse are the secondary impairments that progressively influence movement. For example, most children with cerebral palsy are not born with joint contractures or areas of excessive range (the musculoskeletal system). These develop because of impairments in the neuromuscular system (sustained muscle activity, muscle imbalance, or lack of muscle activity); poor alignment to initiate movement; weakness; poor sensory feedback of movement execution; growth; and other factors. Therefore, joint contractures or areas of excessive range are secondary impairments. For teenagers with cerebral palsy, these contractures or areas of excessive range may be the biggest obstacle to functional independence.

Understanding the development of secondary impairments is extremely important for two reasons. When parents hear the diagnosis of cerebral palsy and the explanation that it is a non-progressive lesion, health care professionals often do not explain clearly what that means. It is true that in CP the lesion itself (the pathophysiology) is presumed not to change. However, the *results* or impairments from this lesion do change, and often some of the child's movement control and function get worse as the child grows. Parents, hearing that cerebral palsy is non-progressive, believe that their child will not get worse. The effects of multiple impairments caused by the lesion, repetition of dysfunctional movements, and a growing, changing child will influence and change the results of the lesion.

The second reason to delineate primary from secondary impairments is that therapists may have a stronger influence on the course of development of these secondary impairments than on the primary impairments. Therefore, an understanding of how secondary impairments develop offers the opportunity to intervene as much as possible before they begin. This requires an understanding of the likely changes that occur in children and adults with cerebral palsy. Those who know and treat only very young children have not had the opportunity to observe and think about changes that occur over time, yet are in the important position of minimizing the formation or development of secondary impairments.

The following systems typically are impaired in cerebral palsy:

- neuromuscular
- sensory and perceptual
- musculoskeletal
- respiratory

Neuromuscular system
Reflexive tone

This is the response to deep tendon reflex testing and to studies of the influence of long and short loop latency responses in posture and movement. Reflexive tone also may include tonic as well as phasic stretch responses.

Muscle activity

This ability depends on information from the CNS to bring about muscle contraction through excitatory impulses and to stop muscle activity by inhibitory information to the alpha motor neuron. Muscle contraction also could cease when excitatory impulses cease. The CNS delivers information to the muscle to contract, continue contraction, or stop contraction. This is a concerted effort of the many functions of many different areas of the CNS working together. A lesion in any part of the CNS can disrupt the delivery of information to the muscle and cause problems initiating muscle activity, keeping it firing when needed, or stopping that firing when movement termination is desired.

Graded agonist/antagonist activity

This involves the ability to grade the activity between cocontraction and reciprocal inhibition. (See Appendix B.)

Muscle synergies

Synergies are groups of muscles working together to produce a desired effect (Lee, 1984). Neuromuscular synergies may be thought of as groups of muscles coordinated by the CNS to constrain intentional action. This means that the CNS has complex mechanisms for selecting and implementing motor strategies through groups of muscles working together in predictable ways to solve functional problems. Predictable timing and ordering, as well as force relationships between muscles controlled by the CNS, help reduce the number of possible movements used to solve functional movement problems.

Many therapists may think of synergies in a negative light, having been taught that a synergy was a primitive or abnormal muscle pattern. However, a synergy is a group of muscles working together to perform a posture or movement. It implies neither good nor bad, right nor wrong.

The child experiencing normal development is able to combine many different muscles together to perform many different postures and movements. The more skilled a movement becomes, the more the muscles work together in precisely timed patterns. Also, the more skilled a movement, the more the child uses only those muscles necessary to the task, thus conserving energy. There is a precise spatial (the ordering of particular muscles or parts of muscles) and temporal (timing) firing of these synergies with skilled function.

Sensory/Perceptual systems
Vision for postural control and movement

Some of the primary impairments in vision are documented in cerebral palsy, such as myopia and retinal detachment that can result from retinopathy of prematurity (Hebbandi et al., 1997). Many believe that at least half of children with CP have visual problems—some estimates go as high as 100% (Duckman, 1987). Primary impairments include ocular motor problems such as strabismus, which interferes with binocular vision and visual fields; ocular problems such as significant refractive errors; and processing impairments such as visual-perceptual dysfunction. Duckman notes that children with CP commonly have difficulty with visual fixation, tracking, and saccadic movements (small, jerky movements of the eyes as they move from one fixation point to another, as in reading). He and others in the field of developmental optometry have been instrumental in developing visual training programs for children with cerebral palsy.

There are other visual problems that develop over time in children with CP that are not as well documented, but are clinically observable. These secondary impairments become just as devastating as the primary impairments and can interfere with any primary impairment remediation or training of visual skills. Children with cerebral palsy often have difficulty lifting and holding up their heads because of primary impairments in the neuromuscular system. This is especially true for those with poor ability to initiate and sustain muscle contraction and poor ability to use cocontraction patterns. Yet the child tries to lift the head anyway. A common finding is that the child uses extension wherever he can manage to recruit it. In babies developing normally, this recruitment of extension also is seen, but to a lesser and more transient extent—the proverbial surprised look of the infant often is a holding with eyebrow raising and forehead muscle recruitment. Part of the extension pattern used is eye extension—upward gaze. This seems to be an easily recruited and easily sustained extension pattern. The result is that the child uses the eyes for postural control, instead of their intended purpose—learning about the environment through vision. This is a disastrous trade-off.

Therapists must be intensely aware of these visual problems, whether coming from the perspective of physical, occupational, or speech therapy. There is a large body of research showing that infants and young children rely on and learn postural control first primarily through use of their visual systems. Learning includes posture (Butterworth & Hicks, 1977; Lee & Aronson, 1974; Shumway-Cook & Woollacott, 1995) and visual awareness of self in relationship to the environment (Bertenthal & Campos, 1987).

Information as feedback

There have been some studies that address problems in proprioceptive, tactile, and vestibular functioning in children with cerebral palsy. These studies primarily look at children with hypertonia, athetosis, and ataxia, and will be addressed in those chapters.

As Lee (1988) points out, people with CNS pathology can show at least two distinct problems in sensory/perceptual function. The threshold for sensory feedback, which often is involved in correcting postural errors, may be abnormal. There can be an abnormally high or low threshold to sensory information, or there can be delays in feedback so that normal error correction never is provided. In children with hypertonia, for example, using treatment techniques that give repetitive tactile and proprioceptive input often results in better motor performance. Perhaps these children have a higher threshold for receiving and processing sensory information. On the other hand, giving organized tactile and proprioceptive input to children with ataxia often yields lesser results in improved motor performance. Children with ataxia are assumed to have profound sensory processing impairments; perhaps their systems cannot perceive and integrate the sensory information provided well enough to correct movement or to learn new motor strategies.

More research is needed in this area. Are these sensory/perceptual impairments primary, secondary, or both? There may be a higher threshold for sensory information coming into the CNS and/or problems interpreting and using this information in children with CP. But there also may be secondary impairments in the sensory systems due to lack of use. When a child moves very little because of neuromuscular impairments, the sensory systems receive very little input and so are *inexperienced*. This was one of the initial concepts developed by the Bobaths that separated their philosophy from other treatment approaches in the 1950s (Bobath & Bobath, 1964; Bobath, B., 1971). There is evidence that sensory receptors adapt adversely to little or no stimulation from the environment, as well as from lack of self-generated movement (Held, 1965). If primary impairments are also part of the picture in children with cerebral palsy, then understanding them more thoroughly will enable us to devise more exact treatment strategies. When secondary impairments are also part of the picture, then this provides therapists another rationale for the earliest possible intervention.

Musculoskeletal system

Several factors influence growth and changes in the skeleton, both positively and negatively. The skeleton changes in response to growth hormones, nutritional factors, and the forces placed on joints and bones (Wolff's law) (LeVeau & Bernhardt, 1984).

The impairments in bony structure seen in children with cerebral palsy are usually secondary. They develop over time for a variety of reasons, including:

1. impact of gravity on a body that is poorly aligned and moves abnormally

2. impact of abnormal muscle contractions on the growth and change of bones

3. lack of variety of movements that children with cerebral palsy make, including weight-bearing postures

Therapists probably can influence the structural changes that occur with growth. We may not be able to eliminate these problems—the forces impacting bony growth and structure work 24 hours a day, and the problems that children with cerebral palsy face are profound and complex. However, a greater understanding of the possible causes of common abnormal bony changes may lead to more effective treatment strategies. Motor control depends not only on the functioning of the nervous system in specific environments, but also on the structure (musculoskeletal system) upon which the nervous system acts.

Some children with CP are born with primary structural bony changes. These may be skeletal deformities that usually are considered an impairment in addition to their cerebral palsy rather than caused by cerebral palsy.

Areas of hypomobility of joints and shortness of muscles usually are secondary impairments. Most children with CP have a normal musculoskeletal structure at birth. This includes some joints and muscles that are not at the adult values of range of motion or muscle extensibility. For example, the pectoralis major muscle is short in a normal newborn compared to a 3-month-old child developing normally or an adult. The muscle goes through a process of lengthening for functional use (Alexander et al., 1993; Bly, 1994). The hip joint is flexed at birth in a child developing normally, so that there is a flexion *contracture* of about 30° (Coon, Donato, Houser, & Bleck, 1975; Haas, Epps, & Adams, 1973). By 6 to 7 months in normal development, the child has full range in the hip joint.

Because there are muscles that do not normally have full extensibility at birth, the therapist treating a child with cerebral palsy must be aware of the muscles that are typically short at birth. The therapist also must be aware that there seem to be developmental processes that typically increase extensibility in these muscles. In addition, the therapist must evaluate atypical increases in tightness of muscles, both those that were tight at birth and those that become tight.

Areas of excessive range of motion, ligamentous laxity, or instability of joints are seen in many children with cerebral palsy. Most of these problems are secondary impairments. Use caution when using *hypermobile* to describe all excesses in muscle length or joint range in children with CP. Hypermobility implies that the ligaments and/or capsule enable range beyond that which is normal for that joint. Because this may not always be the case, a better description may be *excessive range* if the range is increased but not abnormal or *abnormal range* if the movement is aberrant.

Areas of excessive or abnormal range usually are caused by abnormal internal and external stresses on the joint. The therapist's job is to determine what the stresses are. Better yet, the therapist should determine the potential abnormal stresses on a joint and minimize those stresses.

Strength, the ability to produce force, usually is considered part of the musculoskeletal system. Force is exerted through muscle contractions acting on the skeleton. However, strength includes more than the musculoskeletal system. Force production depends on the ability to initiate, sustain, and terminate movement, all of which is regulated by the neuromuscular system. Strength is a neuromusculoskeletal factor in control of posture and movement. Because of this, it often is difficult to determine if lack of strength is a result of abnormal CNS firing to regulate muscle activity, making decreased strength a secondary impairment, or whether the child's system has a primary defect in the ability to produce force in a particular muscle for other reasons (e.g., a metabolic problem).

Children with cerebral palsy often lack sufficient strength to complete functional skills. Much of their insufficient strength appears to be a secondary impairment. Because children with CP often show delayed initiation of muscle activation and difficulty sustaining many of their movements, strength doesn't necessarily develop as the child grows and adds weight. Also, the child with CP initiates muscle activity from poorly aligned joints. Therefore, the muscles are in poor length/tension relationships for producing adequate force to move a joint. Strength tends to remain unused and undeveloped in certain parts of the joint range controlled by the muscle(s).

Respiratory system

Respiratory system muscles, used to support posture and movement, usually are compromised in a child with CP. Easy respiration is vital to the smooth execution of movement and sustaining posture. Many children with cerebral palsy have difficulty maintaining respiration to support posture and movement. A number of these impairments are secondary—they develop over time or there is a failure of development of more mature respiratory patterns from the infant belly-breathing pattern.

The infant breathes primarily with the diaphragm, which sits high in the thoracic ribcage (Alexander, Boehme, & Cupps, 1993). With each inspiration, it contracts, pushing down on the abdominal contents. In the infant, the abdominal muscles are not yet working to oppose this force of the diaphragm, and the belly expands. Thus, the term *belly breathing* is given to this pattern. In addition, the ribcage is elevated and the ribs horizontally positioned, making the ribcage a fairly rigid structure. This is another reason the infant is a belly breather.

During normal development, the baby changes the shape and structure of the ribcage by the muscle activity she is able to recruit, the postures she is able to assume, and the effects of gravity and other outside forces (Alexander et al., 1993; Bly, 1994). The development of spinal extension and the lengthening and use of the intercostal and abdominal muscles are critical in changing the shape of the ribcage. The ribcage can descend from its elevated position to become more mobile so that the child can expand the ribcage when breathing. Using the abdominal muscles resists the action of the diaphragm on inspiration so that the belly does not expand so much. The abdominal muscles also grade exhalation needed for speech.

In children with CP, the ribcage often remains elevated and the spine flexed. Therefore, the ribcage remains immobile and cannot expand with control to increase the volume of air exchange. It also cannot assist in the gradation of exhalation needed for controlled air flow for speech. Often the ribcage changes shape through prolonged positioning, lack of postural muscle activity, or excessive, sustained muscle activity (for example, the barrel chest). These changes are almost always detrimental to respiratory efficiency. In most children with CP, the abdominal muscles fail to be used posturally to support lower trunk stability and to support the ability to shift to the use of ribcage expansion for breathing.

The function of the respiratory system is vital in oxygen exchange. Some children with CP sustain damage to the lungs that interferes with air exchange. This often can be seen in children who are born prematurely. The lungs are damaged and are responsible for inefficient use of respiration (Kelly, 1994; O'Shea et al., 1996). This is a primary impairment—the pathophysiology (some type of lung damage) causes the problem immediately. There may be chronic lung disease subsequently creating a variety of impairments. Therapists must be aware of the limitations that such damage may impose on the child they are treating.

Other systems to consider

The systems detailed previously are those that greatly influence posture and movement, but other systems certainly contribute to posture and movement control and must be considered when evaluating a child's impairments. Systems such as arousal/attention, motivation, cardiorespiratory endurance, nutrition and growth, and skin condition are other systems that should be considered when applicable to the individual child. These systems are considered important sources of impairments that can affect children with cerebral palsy.

Arousal/Attention. Arousal may be defined as physiological readiness for activity. Attention follows this readiness and may be defined as focusing of consciousness or receptivity. Arousal and attention usually are classified as cognitive influences on the control of posture and movement. Thelen, Fisher, Ridley-Johnson, and Griffin (1982) believe that arousal level probably can modify posture and movement. Low arousal levels can interfere with selective attention to environmental stimuli.

Alerting and attention are favored strongly by the tactile and visual systems respectively (Rosenbaum, 1991). Touch alerts us to and vision helps us select what we attend. Children with multiple disabilities, including those with cognitive impairments, visual impairments, and children with traumatic brain injuries or tumors involving the frontal lobes or the brain stem, may have low arousal levels. Children can have difficulties with low attention to environmental stimuli or selectively attending to that which should be important. As therapists, we evaluate these areas as they relate to learning movement (and speech pathologists do so as they relate to language). Bradley (1994) states that in children with normal development, attention is learned, and so the possibility exists that it can be taught in therapy. We also may need to consider what Shumway-Cook and Woollacott (1995) call *attentional costs*. This refers to the need to process information related to a motor task. Therapists add to this attentional cost when giving assistive devices to children.

Motivation. This also is considered a cognitive variable and probably contributes in several ways to the control of posture and movement. Bradley (1994) states that motivation may trigger an activity and shape the consequences of movement. Motivation may influence how quickly we move, the muscle groups we activate, and the attention we give a task.

Cardiorespiratory endurance. In children with cerebral palsy, poor efficiency of the cardiovascular and respiratory systems often are secondary impairments. Poor endurance of these systems, as well as poor endurance of the musculoskeletal system, may be related to primary impairments in the neuromuscular system that compromise efficient muscle contractions, use of efficient muscle synergies, and development of peripheral blood flow. As posture and movement become increasingly difficult to execute for daily activities, it is likely that the development of aerobic capacity is compromised. Researchers are looking into the specific areas of endurance and fitness levels in children with cerebral palsy (Parker, Carriere, Hebestreit, Salsberg, & Bar-Or, 1993; Van den Berg-Emons, van Baak, de Barbanson, Speth, & Saris, 1996).

Digestion and elimination. Children with CP can experience problems with gastroesophageal reflux and constipation (Agnarsson, Warde, McCarthy, Clayden, & Evans, 1993; Heine, Reddihough, & Catto-Smith, 1995). Muscle activity, even smooth muscle, can affect these children and can contribute to these two major digestive tract functions. Abnormal sphincter activity might be treated with medication or surgery. Therapists can influence the function of the digestive system when helping children function in a more upright position and when increasing postural muscle activity in the trunk.

Nutrition and growth. Nutrition can be affected by poor oral motor skills, digestive tract dysfunction, and altered energy requirements for movement. Growth abnormalities may relate to poor nutrition, but also may be due to other factors such as disuse, sensory deficits, decreased blood flow, abnormal growth hormone levels, and abnormal muscle contraction (Coniglio, Stevenson, & Rogol, 1996; Stallings, Charney, Davies, & Cronk, 1993a; Stallings, Charney, Davies, & Cronk, 1993b; Stevenson, Hayes, Cater, & Blackman, 1994; Stevenson, Roberts, & Vogtle, 1995). Therapists must be alert to the problems of poor nutrition and consider its effect on posture and movement. Other team members who can evaluate nutrition and additional medical conditions that contribute to growth may have a great impact on what we are trying to accomplish in our own specialties.

Skin condition. Therapists look at general health and the integrity of children's skin, especially when children are less mobile and less able to shift their weight within a posture, as is seen in many children with CP. Preventing skin breakdown and pain from decreased blood flow is a primary interest. In addition, therapists evaluate and treat scar tissue and healing surgical wounds to minimize loss of range of motion. Many surgical scars cross joints and may contribute to loss of range of motion as scar tissue forms. There also is the possibility of adherence of skin to the superficial tubing of ventriculoperitoneal shunts that children may have.

Typical Posture and Movement Strategies

This section describes the typical development and movements often seen in children with hypotonic, spastic, athetoid, and ataxic cerebral palsy. This information is based on clinical observations and clinical reasoning from evaluation and assessment of the impairments that children with CP typically present. Knowledge of the child's impairments based on research and clinical observations helps the therapist formulate theories as to why a child develops and moves the way he does.

Knowing or theorizing what the impairments are may not give the entire picture of why children function the way they do, however. There has been a recent shift in the therapy literature away from evaluating and treating the impairments to evaluating the impairments, functional limitations, disabilities, and societal limitations, and trying to see the interrelationships of these levels of movement dysfunction to functional outcome. Not everyone is convinced that there is always a direct and linear relationship between the impairments, functional limitations, and disabilities (Jette, 1995). However, the interrelationship of the impairments, both those we are aware of and those that we don't know how to evaluate, often result in predictable functional outcomes. Yet, therapists do not always understand fully all the impairments and how they affect each other.

In the NCMRR disability model (and other disability models), one category that could help bridge the gap between impairments and functional limitations is not described. Several clinicians who use disability models have tried to bridge this gap, naming the category to suit their needs—*composite impairments, multisystem impairments,* and in this text *typical posture and movement strategies.* The category is used to describe an outcome that is presumed to be caused by impairments in several systems that together affect functional outcome, therefore causing functional limitations.

Many pediatric therapists find that there are fairly predictable ways that children with CP develop and learn movement. They can predict how the child is likely to move and what functions are likely to develop based on these posture and movement strategies. For example, consider the problem of lack of head control. This is not an impairment because it can be caused by a combination of impairments in more than one system. It also is not a functional limitation because a functional reason for having head control has not yet been identified. Yet lack of head control is a common developmental problem for children with CP, affecting many functions and leading to many disabilities and societal limitations. The following list may help sort out the causes and effects of lack of head control in a child. (Remember that a lack of head control may be caused by different impairments in different children.)

Possible impairments. Lacks the ability to use and grade the flexors and extensors together for cocontraction as needed; lacks ability to sustain any muscle group for more than several seconds at a time; eyes do not work together well enough to give accurate visual feedback about head position in space; upper cervical extensors are tight and do not allow range into a chin tuck position.

Posture and movement strategies. The head often is held or dropped back in capital extension (head on cervical spine extension) with the eyes looking at the ceiling regardless of the posture in which the child is placed. The child cannot use cervical rotation or a chin tuck to visually search the environment. The cervical flexors, primarily the infrahyoids, are overstretched in this constant posturing of the head, and the hyoid and laryngeal system are not well stabilized posteriorly. This interferes with vocalizations and feeding. In other words, the child lacks head control.

Functional limitations. The child cannot eat solids with texture or drink thin liquids. The child cannot vocalize many sounds. The child cannot visually locate most toys in her environment to initiate play.

Disabilities. The child is on a limited diet and is restricted as to who can feed her. The child cannot communicate with vocalizations or talking. She cannot play with toys, read, or use vision to communicate.

Societal limitations. People do not attempt to communicate with her or try to find a way to understand her wants or needs. She is not given toys to play with or books to look at and is presumed not to understand what is said to her because she does not look at people when they speak to her.

The category of *typical posture and movement strategies* helps bridge the gap between impairments and functional limitations. It helps provide an understanding of how the functional limitations develop and how the impairments interrelate. Because of this, the therapist should have a better understanding of the necessity of identifying impairments and predicting how these impairments may work together to cause future functional limitations and disabilities.

Years ago (and probably frequently today), therapists used this category of *typical posture and movement strategies* as their problem list in their documentation. It was and is common to see a problem list that looks like this:

- lacks head control
- lacks postural control in sitting
- cannot vocalize, other than an "ahh" sound
- doesn't use right arm to play

But a problem list like this doesn't tell the therapist *why* the child cannot do those things. The disability model helps therapists analyze the causes of the problems so that more specific and individualized treatment results. Analyzing the causes of the child's unique posture and movement strategies is the therapist's role and makes the therapist a necessary part of the child's treatment. Anyone can see that the child doesn't use his right arm to play—it doesn't take a therapist to figure that out! What the therapist does that no one else is trained to do is figure out why the child does not use the arm to play (impairments and their effects on each other), and the functional limitations and disabilities that are likely to result as the child gets older because he does not use his right arm to play when he is 8 months old.

Each chapter will examine the interrelationship of many of the impairments suspected to be typical in children with cerebral palsy and predict the outcomes of movement, both on a functional limitation and disability level in children who receive no intervention.

General Treatment Strategies

Treatment involves an organized plan to intervene with the child's impairments, functional limitations, disabilities, and societal limitations to teach a new function. This is where the therapist must assess the child's potential to achieve a skill that without treatment probably would not develop on its own. One way a therapist may assess this situation is to identify the impairments, to reason how they influence each other to limit the ability to develop a skill, and to decide whether treatment can change them enough to help the child develop the skill. The therapist also may identify the functional limitations, disabilities, and/or societal limitations; identify the impairments that contribute to these limitations; and plan strategies to intervene.

One section of each subsequent chapter will provide some basic thought processes and treatment strategies to intervene with the impairments typically seen in children with cerebral palsy. They certainly are not the only way to think and to treat children. Therapists must develop plans and strategies that suit their own personality, strengths, work environment, and degree of support from other team members. These suggestions should give therapists a start in developing their own treatment ideas.

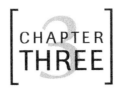

Children With Hypotonia

Pathophysiology

In many infants with signs of possible motor impairments, hypotonia is present at least transiently (Walsh, 1992). This may be because normal postural tone requires normal functioning of the entire nervous system (Fenichel, 1982). This period may last days or years. Other positive signs of CNS dysfunction often emerge eventually. Occasionally, children with CP persist with hypotonia as the major classification. Another possibility is that the child later may be diagnosed with a genetic disorder or other syndrome, for which hypotonia is the primary feature, rather than having cerebral palsy.

Children who have hypotonia that persists beyond early infancy may have involvement of the cerebellar pathways with an enlarged ventricular system seen on neuroimaging (Kuban & Leviton, 1994). Often, the lesion is unknown. Some children with hypotonia may have abnormal neuromuscular outcomes later (Bartlett & Piper, 1993). Those who develop CP may show signs of ataxic, athetoid, or hypertonic cerebral palsy as they grow and mature. However, they may develop for months or even years as hypotonic.

What is hypotonia? Surprisingly, a definition is difficult to find in the literature. *Hypotonia* usually is described as the way a muscle or limb feels when handled. Shumway-Cook and Woollacott (1985) define it as decreased segmental motoneuron pool excitability and pathology of the stretch reflex.

Researchers who study motor control in children with hypotonia see various problems in control and coordination, which are negative signs of CNS damage. Research primarily has been done with children with Down syndrome, a more homogeneous population to study than children with cerebral palsy. Studies also have been done with the muscular dystrophies. Several impairments other than hypotonia (as defined by Shumway-Cook and Woollacott, 1985) have been identified in these studies. For example, in Down syndrome, researchers identified impairments in speed of initiation of movement; more variable synergies to control postural sway, especially proximally; underdamped movement (oscillations at the end point of movement); and decreased joint stiffness with a decreased ability to use cocontraction (Davis & Kelso, 1982).

Children with syndromes such as Prader-Willi, hydrocephalus, and Down syndrome may exhibit many of the characteristics described in this chapter. Often, more definitive information about movement impairments is known, as well as specific pathophysiology of the CNS, in these syndromes. Children with hypotonic CP, like those with all classifications of cerebral palsy, are hard to study because they are more different from each other than alike. However, clinical observations of children with hypotonic CP reveal several common impairments clinically that lead to predictable movement outcomes.

Impairments in Hypotonic Cerebral Palsy

Neuromuscular system

Possible abnormal reflexive tone

There may be decreased segmental motoneuron pool excitability (as defined by Shumway-Cook and Woollacott, 1985), or there may be no evidence of decreased tonic activity (Van der Meche & Van Gijn, 1986). There are depressed deep tendon reflexes (DTRs) in some children. Others may show brisk DTRs (Kuban & Leviton, 1994). Hypotonia cannot be diagnosed based on the type of DTRs elicited.

Difficulties with muscle contraction

Children with hypotonia seem to have a primary impairment of either reaching threshold for muscle fiber firing and/or recruiting enough motor units for initiating movement. They also have difficulty sustaining muscle activity. Therefore, a therapist sees a quick onset of muscle activity which often lacks grading and that lasts only a second or so when the child does initiate movement. Many clinicians describe this as phasic bursts of movement.

Children with hypotonia also do not grade termination of movement well. Because their muscle contractions usually are unsustained, termination often is a cessation of an attempt to sustain movement. If a child with hypotonia can begin to control termination of muscle activity to some extent, termination still is performed quickly as the child cannot grade muscle activity fully. The child's precision and accuracy are affected.

Difficulties grading agonist/antagonist activity

Children with hypotonic cerebral palsy often cannot generate or sustain cocontraction (or graded interaction of the agonist and antagonist) sufficiently for many functional skills. This is a primary impairment.

In children with severe hypotonia, this is seen in all attempts at movement, beginning with an inability to hold the head or limbs against gravity even if placed for them. In more mildly affected children, this problem usually is seen in skills that require sustained, antigravity muscular activity, especially when cocontraction patterns are necessary (e.g., standing on one foot, then hopping repeatedly, or holding the arms in the air long enough to catch a fly ball in the outfield).

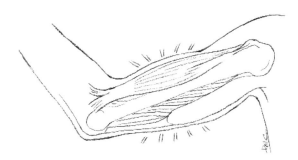

Figure 3.1 Cocontraction is the simultaneous firing of agonist and antagonist muscles around a joint. This results in muscular stability of a joint. In this example, the biceps and triceps of the upper arm stabilize the elbow joint. This may be required for activities such as upper extremity weight bearing in movement transitions such as moving from sit to all fours, carrying a heavy suitcase, lifting a garage door, using a screwdriver, and performing various wrestling holds.

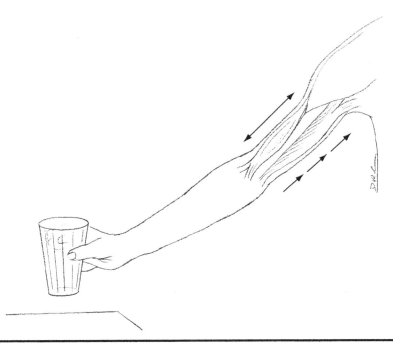

Figure 3.2 Graded movement is the constantly changing relationship of muscle fiber firing between the agonist and antagonist during a movement. Many activities require graded control. For example, placing this glass back on the table without breaking it or spilling its contents requires active lengthening of the biceps with a shortening contraction of the triceps. As the angle of the elbow extension changes, the muscle fiber selection and number of fibers firing changes. This requires constantly updated and changing activation and termination of muscle fiber activity.

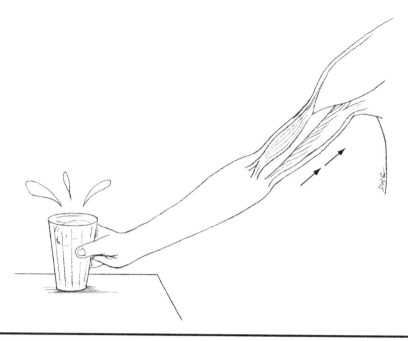

Figure 3.3 This may be one explanation for the lack of graded control in children with hypotonia. They seem to activate the agonist in unsustained contractions with little to no activity of the antagonist. The cup hits the table hard when it is put down. The child also quickly goes to end range of elbow extension to use ligamentous stability instead of graded muscular control to try to control movement.

Limited synergies used to produce posture and movement

The child with hypotonia usually is limited in the synergies combined to produce posture and movement. Therefore, the child's movements lack variety. Clinically, children with pure hypotonia use movement patterns that enable them to use a wide base of support with a low center of mass. It is unclear whether the synergies used are due to the lesion limiting which muscles can be used, or whether certain movement patterns are used and strengthened according to the initial postures of widely based limbs and an inactive trunk. Research is required for both ideas.

The lack of variety of synergies can be a primary impairment. The lesion can cause certain muscles or muscle groups to have difficulty with activation, although there is no evidence of this in the literature specifically in children with hypotonic CP. Studies of children with Down syndrome show that the basic organization of muscle synergies is similar to children without neurological impairments (Davis & Kelso, 1982; Shumway-Cook & Woollacott, 1985). Other studies of children with Down syndrome using ballistic movements also show use of correct synergies (Almeida, Corcos, & Latash, 1994). These studies may lead therapists to look for other primary impairments instead of muscle synergies as a primary impairment in some children with hypotonia.

However, there is evidence that in different types of lesions, even those that seem to be more peripheral than central in origin, postural muscles respond by becoming weak and more dynamic, and phasic muscles respond with overactivity and adaptive shortening (Janda, 1978). If this is so in cerebral palsy, as well as in a variety of other pathophysiologies, the possibility exists that some muscle synergies would be difficult to activate if some of the muscles in the synergy were too tight or weak to respond. This might be considered a secondary impairment—the inability to activate muscle synergies is not due to the lesion limiting the organization of synergies directly, but to the lesion biasing some muscles to become weak and some to become shortened. If length is restored to the muscles with adaptive shortening and the weak postural muscles strengthened, the child may be able to learn to use more functional synergies.

The synergies used by children with hypotonia are very predictable, despite the variety of lesions among them. These children have in common the difficulties of using postural muscles to initiate and sustain antigravity work, and so often substitute more superficial, tight muscles as an attempt to gain upright control. They also use muscle synergies and mechanical stability that enable use of a wide base of support to assist support of positions against gravity. Because their development often is predictable, especially the synergies of posture and movement that they are likely to use, synergies will be covered more fully in the section on posture and movement strategies.

Sensory/Perceptual systems

The child with hypotonia may have both primary and secondary impairments in vision or the use of vision. Primary impairments can include strabismus, loss of visual fields, and refractive errors. Cortical visual impairments also are possible with damage to the many areas of the CNS that process, route, and interpret visual information. The secondary impairments, which can be just as devastating, almost always include the use of the eyes for postural control assistance rather than for exploration of the environment. The eyes are used to help lift and hold the head up. They are not free to visually explore. Moving the eyes to any posture other than upward gaze may cause the child to lose the head position against gravity, especially when the head and cervical spine are in the extreme position of extension.

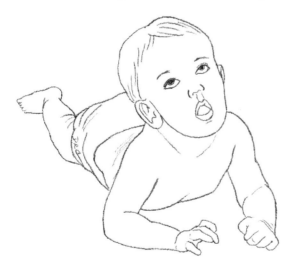

Figure 3.4 This 16-month-old with hypotonia uses upward eye gaze (extension of the eyes) to assist head lift.

Clinical observations suggest that children with hypotonic CP do not use information normally from proprioceptive and tactile systems. Unless they are visually attuned to tactile or joint pressure from the few body movements they make or from objects contacting their bodies, they seem to disregard it. They may use too much or too little force in attempting to complete tasks. If treatment techniques are used to increase the spatiotemporal input of tactile and proprioceptive information to the CNS, many children show appropriate movement or postural responses that they do not make on their own. Perhaps they have a high threshold to firing of these sensory receptors or for perception of this firing. Or it may be simply that the general inactivity of the child with hypotonia causes these systems to be developed poorly to learn the perceptions of body awareness and spatial relationships.

For example, when the therapist uses joint approximation through a well-aligned spine while the child is sitting and trying to reach for an object, the child often is able to recruit more postural trunk muscle activity, making sitting more stable and independent of outside support. The trunk is more active and stable so that the reaching arm has active and dynamic support. The result is quicker, smoother, more accurate reach.

There may be other primary impairments in sensory processing within the CNS that prevent the information from sensory systems from being integrated into motor commands. This may be why some children with hypotonia respond well to organized, meaningful sensory input to help them learn new movements while others do not.

Musculoskeletal system

In children with hypotonia, bony changes are secondary. There can be gradual abnormal changes in the bony structure as the child grows. As bony structure changes, then becomes permanent, it can have an impact on and worsen other primary impairments or lead to other secondary impairments such as skin breakdown.

Children with hypotonia have a poor ability to generate internal forces to oppose gravity and other external forces. Their muscle contractions often are infrequent and unsustained. It is not uncommon for moderately-to-severely affected children to spend months or even years lying down, usually in the supine position. In addition, their initial positions of wide-based limbs and an inactive trunk provide a poor starting position to generate the forces that lead to proper molding of bones.

In the spine and ribcage, profound changes often occur that have the potential to affect major internal organs. Marked abnormalities in spinal curves and ribcage structure develop because of abnormal muscle pull and/or lack of muscle activity on all sides of the trunk, the influence of gravity, the depth and pattern of respiration, as well as genetic and nutritional factors. Children with hypotonia tend to

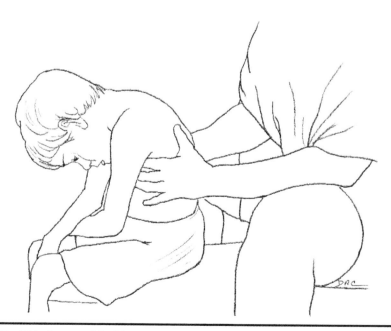

Figure 3.5 This 9-year-old with severe involvement is unable to lift his head. His thoracic spine is severely kyphotic with the postural and superficial extensors overstretched.

Chapter Three

retain and increase the infant kyphosis of the entire spine, except for the cervical area in some who can lift and hold their heads erect. This kyphosis also is seen in very mildly affected children, although to a much lesser extent. The ribcage often is flattened anterior-posteriorly and tends to remain elevated with more horizontal alignment of the ribs and flaring of the inferior ribs laterally and/or anteriorly.

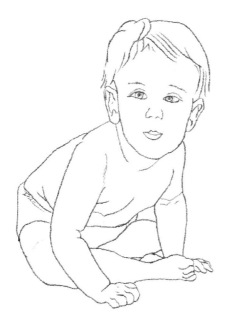

Figure 3.6a At 16 months, this toddler can sit supported, propped on her arms, for brief periods. One reason she cannot sit alone is the lack of active trunk extension. Her thoracic spine is mildly kyphotic.

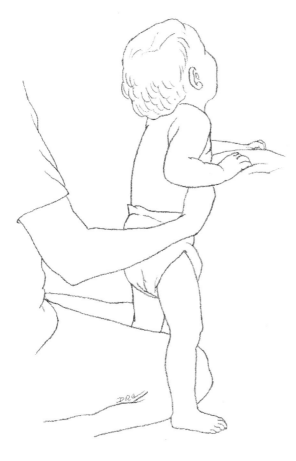

Figure 3.6b In standing, the 16-month-old shows the mild kyphosis through her thoracic and lumbar spine. She attempts to use cervical extension to help herself stand erect, but this is ineffective due to the cervical spine's distance from the hips and center of mass, and due to the lack of extension throughout the trunk and lower extremities necessary for standing.

The other common bony changes seen in children with hypotonia are at the hip and shoulder joints. These are secondary impairments because they develop over time. The possibility exists in the hip that the acetabulum could remain shallow with the femoral head flattened because of late and insufficient weight bearing. This can result in subluxation and dislocation. Again, although the studies of children with hypotonia do not look specifically at children with hypotonic CP, these problems are cited (Diamond, Lynne, & Sigman, 1981; Shea, 1990). Clinically, a number of children with hypotonia and athetosis sublux their shoulders, usually inferiorly or anteriorly. This can be due to laxity of the ligaments and/or capsule or it can be due to prolonged positioning. Hips and shoulders have the possibility of subluxing/dislocating anteriorly when the limb is abducted and externally rotated, then pressed distally against a surface (usually in supine) while the head and trunk extend. This would be compounded if the ligaments also are lax.

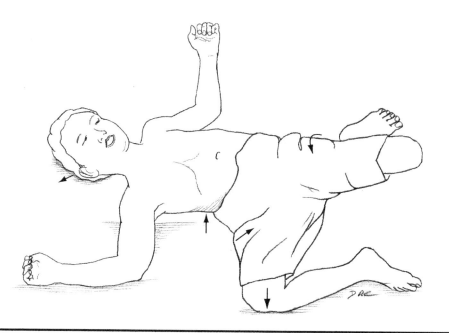

Figure 3.7 This 4-year-old developed for several years with severe hypotonia before he also showed athetoid movements. As he began to use asymmetrical extension in supine to push against the floor, he placed stress on the anterior shoulder joint *(see arrows for direction of forces)*. The forces that place stress on the anterior shoulder joint, combined with the underlying poor muscular activity and ligamentous integrity, can lead to anterior shoulder joint dislocation.

Children with hypotonic CP often develop further tightness in muscle groups that are typically in shortened positions from birth. This could be considered a secondary impairment because it worsens over time. The muscles that typically remain short or shorten over time are the superficial muscles, two-joint muscles, and muscles that are considered phasic as opposed to more postural in their intended function. These muscles may try to substitute for postural muscles when the postural muscles are unable to function against gravity. Some examples of these are: latissimus dorsi, scapular elevators, upper cervical erector spinae, lumbar erector spinae, pectorals, and hamstrings.

Other muscles or muscle groups tighten in response to the child's constant, unchanging position. This is seen in severely involved children who lie in one or two positions for many hours. It also is seen in more mildly involved children who maintain a slightly wide base of support in any position and tend to move their trunks in the sagittal plane only. Examples of these are: intercostals, quadratus lumborum, hip abductors, and hip external rotators.

Children with hypotonic CP are well known for areas of joint laxity or excessive range. It is unclear whether this is a primary or secondary impairment. In children with Down syndrome, the problem is at least partially a primary impairment because there seems to be a collagen defect that causes ligamentous laxity (Gajdosik & Ostertag, 1996). In all children with hypotonia, however, at least some of their excessive range develops over time because of abnormal stresses on the joints from constant positions or movements. These areas of excessive range then would be secondary impairments and at least partially preventable if the child avoided those stresses.

Speculation may apply as to which areas of excessive range are primary and which are secondary, but some seem to be present initially, which leads to the belief that they are primary. These include finger and thumb hyperextension, elbow hyperextension, knee hyperextension, and excessive hip movements in all ranges. Also, some children with hypotonia show a tendency toward shoulder joint dislocation from birth.

Other excessive or abnormal joint movements develop over time, and so are at least partially secondary in nature. Examples of these include shoulder or hip dislocation that is not seen at birth or shortly after, pronation of the feet, and sometimes a sharp extension with or without abnormal lateral movement at the thoracolumbar junction of the spine.

The child with hypotonic CP may or may not have a problem with strength, which is the ability of the muscle to produce force. Clinically, it can be very difficult to separate strength from neuromuscular impairments. Is the problem that the child cannot generate sufficient force under any condition or that he can't generate it fast enough or sustain it long enough for certain functions due to neurological processes that activate or sustain muscle firing? In children with Down syndrome, an amino acid deficiency seems to be at least partially responsible for delayed initiation of movement (Davis & Kelso, 1982). However, these children often are able to generate sufficient and even excessive grip forces when given enough time, leading to the conclusion that normal strength is possible for them (Cole, Abbs, & Turner, 1988).

The child with hypotonia often learns early that she can use the close-packed positions of joints to *stabilize* them to substitute for sustained or midrange joint positions using muscle activity. Close-packed positions of the joints are biomechanically stable because, in these positions, the joint surfaces are most congruent. This skeletal stability is used to substitute for muscular control and strength, thereby preventing the development of strength throughout the entire range of joint motion. Also, children with hypotonia often do not develop the strength of many muscle groups because they assume positions of a wide base of support. These positions place many muscle groups in poor length-tension relationships for activation and use for postural stability or body segment movement.

Respiratory system

Children with hypotonic cerebral palsy usually show shallow respiration with a belly-breathing pattern. Often their ribcages show flattening anterior-posteriorly with lateral rib flaring of the lower ribcage on inspiration. The ribcage is elevated. Although some of these respiratory problems may be primary impairments, most of them probably are secondary.

Belly breathing relies on a simple pattern of movement only. The diaphragm contracts relatively unopposed or unassisted, although in normally developing children the musculature of the ribcage helps hold the shape of the ribcage. The abdomen expands with inspiration as the diaphragm descends. The ribcage is immobile or moves very little in the lower ribs. This is the pattern that is seen in newborns (Alexander et al., 1993). The child with hypotonia shows ribcage changes influenced primarily by position and gravity, not by internal musculature forces. The child also has difficulty using more complex synergies of movement to control respiration.

Many functions require more variety in control of respiration. For example, speech requires expansion of the ribcage while musculature supports the ribs. Speech is produced on controlled exhalation, with graded force produced in the diaphragm, abdominal muscles, intercostals, and sometimes the accessory respiratory muscles.

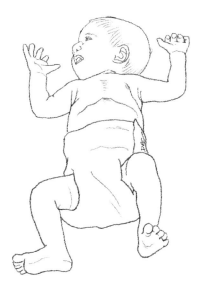

Figure 3.8a This 10-day-old girl shows the normal belly-breathing pattern. Her ribcage is elevated in her trunk, her pectorals and intercostal muscles are tight, and her horizontally positioned ribs give her ribcage a rigid structure. Therefore, thoracic expansion during breathing, even when crying, is minimal. However, a newborn's ribcage has one advantage over an older child's with the same structure—the ribs are more cartilaginous than the older child's and offer some minimal expansion during respiration.

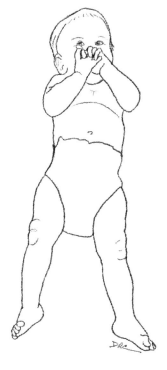

Figure 3.8b This 16-month-old uses belly breathing only to control respiration. Note that the base of her ribcage sits high in her trunk. She retains the infant's structure as her ribs become more osseous.

Chapter Three

Typical Posture and Movement Strategies
Head, neck, tongue, eyes

The child with hypotonia often can rely only on phasic bursts of muscle activity to lift the head. This is true in all positions—whether held upright against a caregiver's shoulder or lying prone, in supported sitting or standing. Because of this, the child compensates, if possible, with musculoskeletal integrity to substitute for sustained, graded movement. This means that the child will use ligamentous, muscular, and capsular length to control and limit movement as well as approximating body segments against each other to limit movement. In addition, the child may show a high threshold to perceiving somatosensory information, making the feedback of the gradation of movement difficult to regulate.

In the cervical spine, the child with hypotonia lifts the head with extension, a movement used by any child to first lift the head. But instead of holding it—even briefly—the head either falls forward or back. If it falls forward against the surface it first lifted from, the child cannot learn anything new visually or posturally. However, if it falls backward with the occiput resting against the upper thoracic spine, the child can see something and is keeping his head up. This works especially well in an infant with hypotonia trying to learn head control because of the relatively large head in comparison to the body and the more rounded thoracic spine seen in infants. The child's head can rest against the spine without falling back very far. Often the child learns that shoulder elevation (a position of the shoulder complex seen in all infants) is a good substitute for cervical control. The child simply rests the head between the two elevated shoulders without needing any more than an initial, short-lived burst of cervical extension to lift the head.

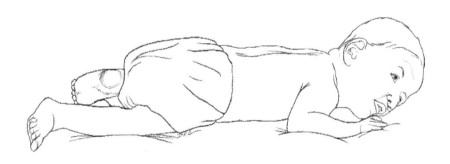

Figure 3.9 This newborn lifts his head using cervical extension.

This method of holding the head up has severe implications and can cause many secondary impairments:

- lack of development of active capital flexion on an extended cervical spine (chin tuck)

- overlengthening of the cervical flexors, especially because, as the child grows older, the head becomes relatively smaller in relationship to the body, and therefore has to fall back farther to rest on the spine

- a shift in the position of the laryngeal system

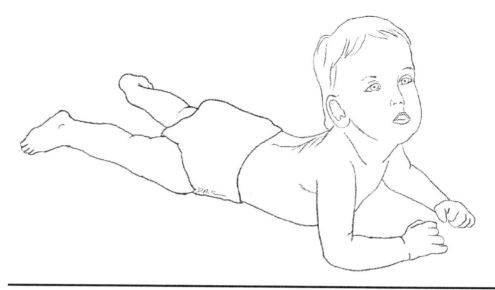

Figure 3.10 Th is child with hypotonia lifts her head using cervical and upper thoracic extension with some weight bearing on her arms. Her mid-thoracic area through most of her lower extremities are resting against the support surface. She is not showing an ability to use her cervical flexors to tuck her chin. Her eyes look upward.

- use of upward visual gaze to help lift the head, and then the inability to move the eyes into any other position once the head is resting back on the spine

- passive opening of the jaw with tongue retraction and overstretching of the facial muscles

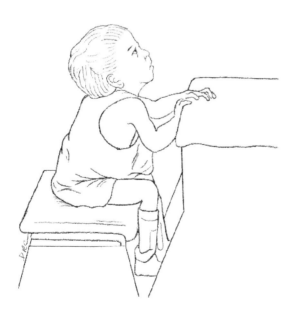

Figure 3.11 This young child rests his head back on his spine after lifting it with extension. Note his use of shoulder complex elevation to provide skeletal stability for his head. His cervical flexors and laryngeal system are stretched. His eyes look up and his jaw is beginning to open.

If the child cannot lift the head at all, or lifts it and it falls forward again, the following secondary impairments may develop:

- lack of development of an active chin tuck

- overlengthening of the cervical and upper thoracic extensors, especially as the child grows older and the relatively smaller head can drop down even farther

- partial obstruction of the airway

- little use of vision to learn about the world

- passive opening of the jaw, although perhaps not as much as if the head were back, with an increased likelihood of drooling

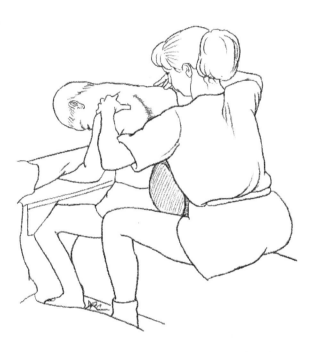

Figure 3.12 This teenager often hangs his head forward. His cervical and thoracic extensors are in an over-lengthened position. He is only able to look at his lap.

Functionally, the child with hypotonia has limitations that likely will result from the primary and secondary impairments. The child probably will be unable to visually explore himself, the environment, and other people in all fields of vision. Depth perception likely will be compromised because its development relies on convergence of the eyes and self-initiated movement through space. The child will have difficulties with feeding and sound production because of the alignment of the oral and laryngeal structures, as well as the inactivity of the muscles responsible for these activities. The child may learn to use tongue retraction to attempt to hold the head up and to control the oral area because these muscles are tight at birth. Breathing might be compromised. The child's cervical spine will not develop the ability to move in all planes in order to orient the head to visual, proprioceptive, vestibular, and auditory information.

A variety of disabilities can result from the various problems in head, neck, tongue, and eye control. For example, an infant's disabilities may include not being able to play with toys, vocally interact with her mother, or feed from the breast or bottle well enough to get adequate nutrition. A 6-year-old's disabilities may be that she cannot learn to read, chew food, or talk at age level. A more mildly involved 10-year-old who shows these same impairments but to a lesser extent may be unable to visually track a moving ball to swing at with a bat, may articulate poorly and therefore be poorly understood, and may be unable to keep all of his food in his mouth when eating. A severely involved 16-year-old may be unable to eat orally, to use vision to discern familiar people (perhaps from primary as well as secondary visual impairments), or to vocalize for any communicative needs.

Thoracic spine, ribcage, and upper extremities

Children with hypotonic cerebral palsy start their postural control and movements from some of the same positions that infants developing normally do. This includes a rounded thoracolumbar spine, elevated ribcage with elevated scapulae, clavicles and shoulders, internally rotated shoulders, flexed elbows and hands, and pronated forearms. The ribs are close together and horizontally oriented. The ribcage is round, with the anterior-posterior and transverse diameters equal (Alexander et al., 1993; Bly, 1994). The infant is a belly breather because of the immobile ribcage, but the cartilaginous ribcage has some give to it as the infant breathes.

Children with hypotonia begin attempts to lift the head at various chronological ages, but tend to start out with a body that is more wide-based in the extremities (the limbs are abducted away from the midline) and with more of the trunk contacting the surface if laid prone or supine.

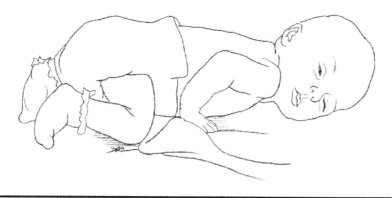

Figure 3.13   This newborn lies prone with weight on her cheek, chest, hands, knees, and toes. Her limbs are close to her body.

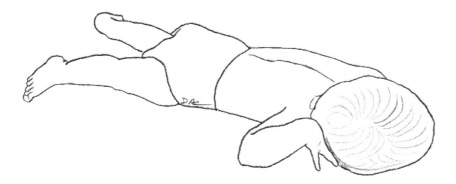

Figure 3.14   The child with hypotonia lies prone with most of the anterior surface of her trunk against the support surface. Her head is rotated so that her ear and cheek rest against the surface. Her limbs abduct.

Chapter Three

As the child with hypotonia tries to lift the head and maintain it upright in any position, the head usually falls back onto the rounded spine. The elevated shoulder complex, including the clavicle, scapula, and shoulder, can enhance stability by enabling the head to be placed between the elevated shoulders, providing some lateral stability. It is extremely important to note that when the child uses elevation of the shoulder complex, shoulder (glenohumeral) joint extension and internal rotation are strongly favored. In fact, it is difficult to assume other positions at the shoulder. Consequently the child suspends the weight of the head and trunk on the integrity of the ligaments and other soft tissue tightnesses of the shoulder complex. This substitutes for using sustained or intermittent muscular control to hold the trunk's antigravity postural control and to keep shoulders active in weight bearing.

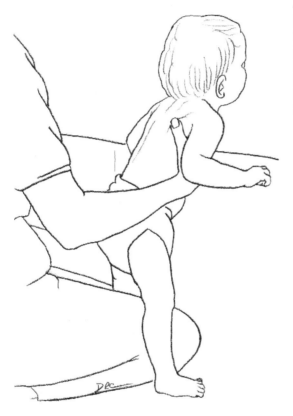

Figure 3.15 In standing, the child with hypotonia retains the elevated position of her shoulder complex as she uses cervical extension to lift her head. She can then allow her head to rest against her upper thoracic spine.

In normal development, there appears to be a strong relationship between gaining active spinal extension and weight bearing of the upper extremities. As the head lifts and holds antigravity and turns from side to side, spinal extension mobility increases. Then, as the arms push actively down into a surface, they aid in lifting the chest up (Alexander et al., 1993; Bly, 1994). In children with hypotonia, part or all of this development is missed. Therefore, the thoracic spine tends to remain rounded, and the relatively inactive arms stay in shoulder (glenohumeral) extension and internal rotation, usually with abduction. The entire shoulder complex elevates, pulling or keeping the ribcage up with it. Therefore, shoulder complex muscles that elevate maintain or increase their tightness, as do the strong internal rotators of the shoulder (latissimus dorsi and pectorals). Because there can be no controlled lateral movement of the trunk from this position of the head and upper extremities, the ribcage not only remains elevated, but the intercostal muscles that are supposed to lengthen with controlled lateral movements cannot do so. The ribcage also may mold with position and gravity to a more flattened anterior-posterior diameter.

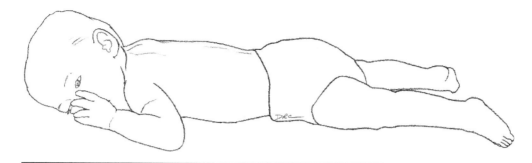

Figure 3.16 This child with hypotonia shows the elevated position of the shoulder complex, an elevated ribcage, and little to no activation of antigravity postural control, all of which compromise the development of muscular length and support of the child's ribcage.

When the child is placed or held in supported sitting, she uses what she has learned about controlling or not controlling her head against gravity. Although this may develop mobility in the upper and/or lower cervical spine, the thoracic spine remains inactive. In sitting, the thoracic spine succumbs to the effects of gravity and its initial bias toward flexion (rounding). Because the ribcage is elevated, the rounding of the spine may enable some mobility between the ribs posteriorly, but not anteriorly or laterally. Therefore, the extensor muscles of the trunk become over-lengthened while the flexor and lateral musculature shortens. In this position, the scapulae abduct and elevate with forward tipping. If the arms abduct, the scapulae are likely to rotate upwardly. If they stay more by the side, then they may be in a position of more downward rotation. The weight of the upper body is loaded onto the diaphragm and abdominal contents, which may make breathing, digestion, and elimination more difficult.

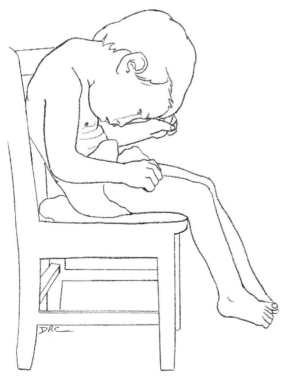

Figure 3.17a This 4-year-old boy shows severe over-stretching of his cervical and thoracic extensor muscles. His upper body weight is loaded onto his diaphragm, which compromises respiration in addition to the compromise in respiration caused by his elevated ribcage.

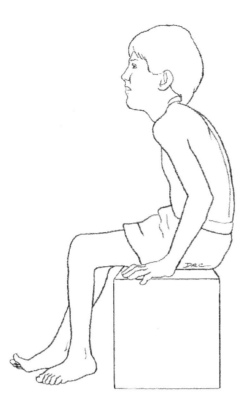

Figure 3.17b This 6-year-old shows less thoracic rounding, but still will compromise respiratory depth due to the weight of his upper body loading onto his diaphragm.

In a more mildly involved child, many of these same positions are present to a lesser extent. There may be some ability to lift and hold the head erect with neuromuscular control, but an inability to sustain it for long, so that it eventually rests against the spine. There also may be an ability to develop the shoulder complex activity of pushing down against a surface for short periods of time, thereby helping to develop active shoulder complex control and assisting with lifting the chest and spinal extension. As the chest lifts higher, the shoulders might move into more flexion, toward external rotation and horizontal adduction. But this child often needs a rest and will assume a position of more thoracic rounding with shoulder complex elevation.

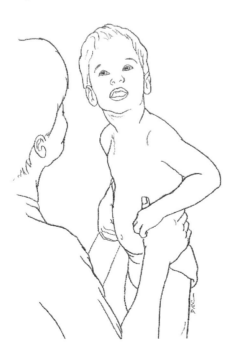

Figure 3.18 This boy is able to stand with assistance to his lower trunk and hips. He occasionally stands erect with fairly normal alignment, but quickly becomes fatigued and collapses into thoracic flexion with his shoulders following into elevation, extension, and internal rotation. He overuses cervical extension in an attempt to remain standing.

Children With Hypotonia

Functionally, the child with hypotonia has many limitations, as he is unable to develop more thoracic extension and graded shoulder mobility. First, the arms are used to substitute for trunk control—they prop with the integrity of the musculoskeletal system, using ligamentous integrity and close-packed positions of the joints where possible to assist the child to be more upright. This can occur in any position the child is placed in. Therefore, the child gives up use of the hands for exploration. In a more mildly affected child, this is seen at least some of the time. It is a tremendous sacrifice for the arms to be used for postural support rather than reaching and exploring.

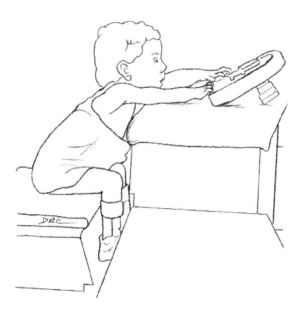

Figure 3.19a This 2-year-old needs his arms supported on the tabletop because he cannot use enough postural trunk control to sit erect. Although he can grab the toy with his fingers from this position, he does not have other options for reach and grasp.

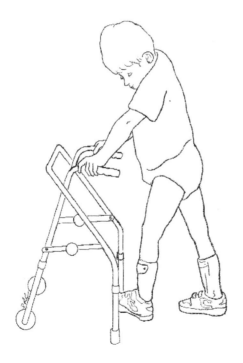

Figure 3.19b This 6-year-old *locks* his elbows into hyperextension as he pushes his walker. This joint position enables him to substitute joint integrity for neuromuscular control. The forward movement of his walker is poorly graded.

Next, the child's respiratory system is compromised—she has not developed the mobility in the ribcage that enables expansion between ribs anteriorly and laterally. The child may further compromise expansion of the abdomen for belly breathing by either lying on the belly in prone or loading the diaphragm with the weight of the upper body when more upright. It is not unusual for a child with severe involvement be comfortable only in supine, probably because of the ease of belly breathing in this position compared with other positions.

When the arms are used to prop with, rather than to reach and explore, the child may never see them. Therefore, visually guided and directed reaching may be affected and limited functionally. If the child moves very little, as seen in many children with hypotonia, poor development and use of all sensory systems for feedback of movement may result and severely compromise learning skilled movement.

Imagine a variety of resulting disabilities. A 2-year-old child with severe involvement who cannot lift or hold his head up likely will have a very kyphotic thoracic spine with overlengthened spinal extensors, arms that bear very little weight, and an elevated, immobile ribcage. Therefore, we can speculate that his disabilities may include the inability to assume or maintain any antigravity posture such as sitting, standing, and walking; an inability to play with most toys, feed himself, or perform any activities of daily living (ADLs); and the inability to use breath support for most vocalizations used for communication. He also will be unable to use gestures, facial expressions, or visual engagement for communication.

A 6-year-old girl with moderate involvement can hold her head erect for short periods, primarily with the superficial cervical extensors. Her thoracic spine is mildly rounded in prone and standing and more rounded in sitting. She can use her arms to reach and manipulate only if sitting or standing with a wide lower extremity base of support or with adaptive equipment supporting her trunk. Otherwise, she must use her arms to help support her trunk in antigravity postures. She is a belly breather with some lateral flaring of the ribs distally. She can speak in short phrases with a limited vocabulary using a soft, whispery voice. Her disabilities may include the inability to walk independently, to write fast enough to keep up with her schoolwork, to use a spoon to eat with, or to communicate with people other than those with whom she is very familiar.

A 16-year-old boy with mild involvement shows a forward-positioned head with capital extension, a mildly rounded spine with slight shoulder complex elevation, abducted and winging scapulae, and shallow respiration with a sunken-appearing chest. His disabilities may include the inability to keep up with his peers when running, the inability to type on the computer fast enough to complete classroom assignments, and cognitive/language deficits that limit his academic abilities. Societal limitations (handicaps) are primarily poor acceptance by some of his peers for the different way he runs, talks, and eats, and his placement in special education.

Lower trunk

In the child with hypotonia, several impairments lead to poor stabilization of the lower trunk with muscular control. Children with hypotonia usually assume two common postures. The first is that many children simply continue the rounding (kyphosis) of the thoracic spine into the lumbar spine. This flexion, or forward bending of the spine, is an unstable position when viewed simply from a biomechanical standpoint: The facet joints are in an open-packed position (a position where the joint surfaces are not congruent—they are not at a place where they fit together, and the joint capsule is on a stretch). This unstable position of the joints requires much more muscular effort for stability than does the close-packed position (extension). The primary impairment that leads to this position is neuromuscular—the poor ability to initiate and sustain muscular activity, especially with the more postural muscles, and the poor ability to use cocontraction. The secondary impairments that result can be lack of strength development in the lower trunk muscles, overstretching or tightness of muscles depending on the posture assumed, and bony deformity from a constant position of the lower trunk.

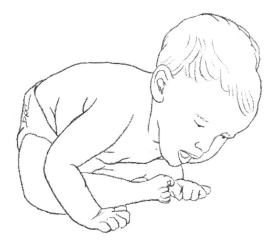

Figure 3.20 This 16-month-old attempts to hold herself up in a prop-sitting position. Her trunk extension, as well as her shoulders and elbows, do not exert or sustain enough force to hold her erect. Lack of trunk activity causes her to try to rely on her arms to stay erect; she is, however, unsuccessful in this attempt.

The second position these children assume is one of sharp upper lumbar extension (even though the thoracic spine is kyphotic, it is not as kyphotic as in the child who rounds the entire spine). When used, this position is usually seen when children are in prone or when they stand. Again, it seems to be a biomechanical (musculoskeletal) system issue. By assuming upper lumbar extension passively, the child gives that area of the spine mechanical stability, often at the expense of not moving at all in the lower trunk. Rather, the child compensates with movement in the head and upper body or the hips. This is very energy costly, as will be described later.

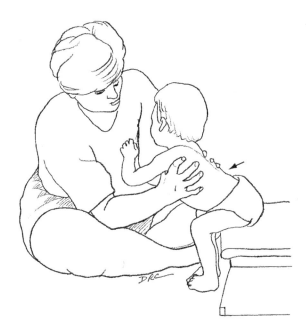

Figure 3.21 This child is assisted to move from sit to stand by his mother. As she helps him bring his weight over his feet prior to standing up, his spine moves into end range extension in the cervical and upper lumbar *(see arrow)* areas.

Which child assumes which position? Although it is never a certainty, most children who use little activity in the upper trunk area to control movement, but rather fall into gravity, simply continue the flexion into the lumbar area. They tend to be children with more severe involvement of their neuromuscular systems—those who cannot initiate or sustain muscular activity most of the time. The upper lumbar extension usually is seen in children who have been able to use at least cervical extension, sometimes with an ability to use some scapular adduction to assist the extension lower in the thoracic spine. However, they do not control with the deeper postural flexors and extensors or with cocontraction or graded interaction of flexors and extensors throughout the body, and they do not use flexion well in the lower trunk. Rather, these children use strong flexion at the hips to try to substitute for stability of the lower trunk with the abdominal muscles. Strong hip flexion, as well as breath holding and tightness in the diaphragm (which attaches to the lumbar spine), may be what helps the child assume this position of upper lumbar extension, resulting in an anterior pelvic tilt. It is not uncommon for a child who uses this position to use it only in prone, W-sitting, and standing, then sink into lumbar flexion when long, chair, or tailor sitting. In none of these positions are the flexor and extensor muscles working together to control and stabilize the lower trunk. Extension is used in standing because the body is relatively more extended throughout, and flexion is used in sitting because the flexion position of the spine and hips is greater here. The child falls into these positions biomechanically because her body has found that this is the only way it has stability.

With the trunk in either flexion throughout the thoracolumbar spine or thoracic flexion with upper lumbar extension, the position of the facet joints at either extreme does not enable the biomechanical advantage of using rotation. Because rotation is difficult from the neuromuscular standpoint anyway, requiring more cooperation through cocontraction of flexors and extensors and timing of these muscles working together, the child with hypotonia has yet another reason to prefer either end-range flexion or extension positioning. However, the center of mass often is controlled through trunk rotation to conserve energy in movement in people without disabilities. When rotation cannot be used, the trunk and often the entire body must use compensatory movements to try to move and change position. These movements can occur in the sagittal or coronal plane (flexion and extension or lateral flexion), but result in a large change in the center of mass and are therefore very energy costly. There is extensive research in gait analysis to show that trunk movements in all three planes are necessary for conserving energy (Krebs, Wong, Jevsevar, Riley, & Hodge, 1992; Thorstensson, Carlson, Zomlefer, & Nilsson, 1982). Flexors and extensors of the lumbar spine work in synergy to stabilize the spine during lower limb movement (Dofferhof & Vink, 1985; Hodges & Richardson, 1997; Perry, 1992).

The abdominal muscles are the muscles that primarily control the anterior surface of the lower trunk. In children with hypotonia, the abdominal muscles are inactive and do not fulfill the role of stabilizing the lumbar spine or the ribcage on the pelvis except for an often tight rectus abdominus which pulls the xyphoid process of the sternum closer to the symphysis pubis and can contribute to more thoracic kyphosis. Abdominal inactivity is of particular interest because it is seen in all types of cerebral palsy and in many other pathologies, even those that do not appear to be of central nervous system origin. Why? Although there is no definitive answer, the explanation appears to be that in injury, postural muscles become weak and inactive and mover muscles tend to become tight (Janda, 1978). The abdominal obliques and transverse abdominus primarily are postural muscles.

The primary impairments of a child with hypotonia include a poor ability to initiate, sustain, and grade termination of the abdominal muscles. The child also has difficulty using any cooperative effort between the lower trunk flexors and extensors.

Secondary impairments of poor respiratory control for breathing while moving and for speech result. Lack of muscular stabilization in the lower trunk is always a problem for children with hypotonia, even for those with the mildest involvement.

It is not uncommon for children with hypotonia to try to generate trunk stability for more skilled movements by holding their breath. The breath holding substitutes for postural muscle activity and joint stability.

In summary, the functional limitations resulting from the combination of impairments are the further compromise of the respiratory system that started with impairments in the upper body and the loss of the ability to control the center of mass efficiently.

Disabilities that result have to do primarily with these two functional limitations. A severely involved 12-year-old may be unable to coordinate swallowing and breathing for eating. This, in addition to problems with the oral phase of feeding, cause him to be unable to eat orally. He also may be unable to cough effectively and can suffer from frequent respiratory infections leading to hospitalization.

A 2-year-old with moderate involvement is unable to sit on the floor independently, although she can sit on a small wooden chair. She walks with a walker but cannot walk independently. She cannot climb stairs, even with assistance of an adult. She can sit in a wooden chair independently, but cannot eat with utensils, as she needs both arms to support herself. She substitutes support with her arms for the control her lower trunk should give her when sitting. For that same reason she is unable to do simple undressing activities. She speaks or vocalizes only in short bursts of sound and, therefore, has the disability of poor intelligibility and lack of age-level phrase length. She cannot vocalize or talk when she is trying to change positions.

A 4-year-old with mild to moderate involvement walks and runs independently, but cannot climb steps without use of a rail. He tires easily during outings and cannot keep up with community level mobility typical of 4-year-olds. He cannot cut with scissors as he is just starting to be able to lift both hands from a surface for bilateral skills when sitting. He cannot do any of his dressing in standing and sits for all of his toileting. He talks slowly and unintelligibly to unfamiliar people.

The pelvic girdle and lower extremities

The two functions of the lower extremities—to provide mobility through space from a stable trunk and to be an active, stable base of support—are compromised in children with hypotonia. Such children often try only one function for their lower extremities—stability with a very wide base. They can assume this position because they usually have the mobility to do so, especially in their hip joints which abduct and externally rotate into greater range than in infants with normal development. They want this very wide base because it often can try to substitute for an unstable trunk. The reason it is not always successful is that their base of support is usually inactive instead of active (mechanical rather than dynamic). Any base of support used in any posture needs to be active—muscles contract to hold us on the support surface and are prepared to contract as needed during weight shifting.

The base of support used by many children with hypotonia is so large that it mechanically blocks movement from other parts of the body, even if those movements are possible for the child or easily within the possibilities of her learning.

The wide base and activity of the lower extremities varies in children with hypotonia according to the severity of their lesion and impairments. However, even in the most mildly involved child, this wide base is present in some postures and movements and interferes with more skilled movements.

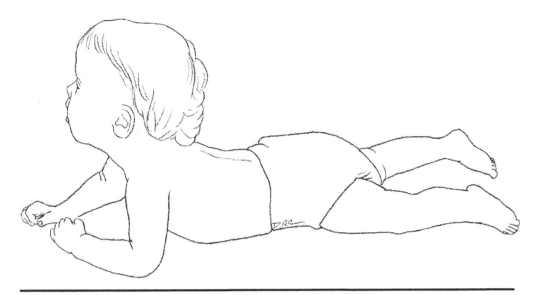

Figure 3.22a In prone, this child has a wide base of support due to abduction of the upper and lower limbs. This limb abduction prevents lateral and rotational movements of the trunk, even if the child has the capability of producing those movements.

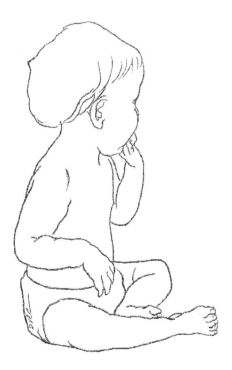

Figure 3.22b Here, the same child is able to sit when placed. She has enough trunk extension to align her head over her trunk and has control of cervical rotation. Her hips are widely abducted and externally rotated. This position of the legs will prevent rotation further down the thoracic spine as well as weight shifting from hip to hip, even if she is capable of producing these movements.

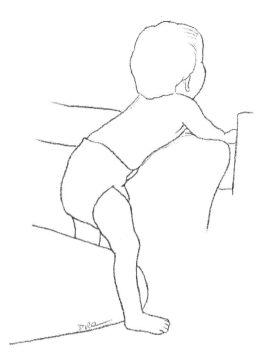

Figure 3.22c In supported standing, the child uses a wide base of support to attempt to control herself against gravity. This may enable her to extend her trunk, hips, and knees, but will not enable her to incorporate trunk lateral movements, trunk rotation, or controlled hip abduction and adduction into sidestepping.

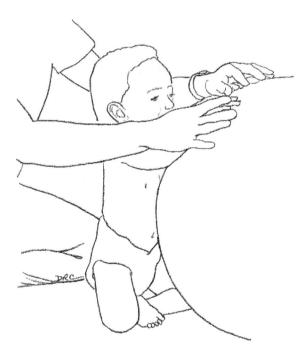

Figure 3.23 This child is being asked to move up to standing from the floor. He keeps his hips in wide abduction with external rotation (he started from a tailor-sitting posture), and cannot actively rotate or laterally flex in his trunk to assist movement of his legs underneath him.

Some of the previous illustrations show various functional limitations that result from the use of the lower body as a very wide base of support only. Again, the limitations include the poor ability to change positions and the poor ability to use the legs for controlled movement while the trunk holds the center of mass stable. Therefore children with hypotonia often don't move much or they use so much energy to move that they are limited in the duration and distance that they can move.

We can imagine some of the resulting disabilities. A 5-year-old with severe hypotonia uses a very wide base of support in prone and supported sitting. Although he already has severe impairments in the upper body that do not enable him to hold his head erect or use his arms, he has no choice but to use his legs as a wide base to make him feel secure when he feels at all threatened about loss of support of his position. The insecurity may be due in part to lack of development of position sense from a lack of self-initiated movement. Another secondary impairment is contractures of the hip flexors, abductors, external rotators, and hamstrings. The limitation of using his lower body as a wide base of support only does not enable him the possibility of movement transitions. Therefore, he has no independent mobility at all—no rolling, crawling, or movement in and out of sitting or standing.

A 13-year-old with mild hypotonia can walk, run, jump, and climb stairs. But she cannot play soccer because she gets short of breath so easily and fatigues due to energy-inefficient movement. She also cannot ride a bicycle or hike with her family.

A 10-year-old with moderate hypotonia can walk, but cannot run, climb stairs with no rail, negotiate curbs, or walk with his class through a museum on a field trip.

General Treatment Strategies

When working with children with hypotonia, start problem solving by looking at the alignment the child uses when assuming postures and executing any movements she is capable of. This helps assess several things at once. Looking at the biomechanics of the child's abilities and inabilities lets the therapist know how much the child's postural control and movement are based purely on muscle length-tension relationship to the joints she is trying to move. Often, simply changing alignment to enable a more efficient length-tension relationship of muscles around a joint provides the child the capability to move, especially if the child is supported initially in other areas of her body for stability and to recruit functional postural synergies.

Another reason to look at alignment first is to try to understand the likely neuromuscular control that the child has or doesn't have. Can he hold up his head? How? Could he hold up his head if his spine were more extended? Hold his spine more erect for him and see. If he can, maybe the control of flexion and extension at the cervical spine isn't so bad. If the control of the cervical spine improves when the position of the trunk is changed, then it is more certain that the head extension is a compensation for lack of spinal extension. Also, look at the wide-based posture of the limbs and at the trunk control to see if the limbs have to remain wide-based because this child cannot control his trunk in all three planes in his current posture.

Looking at alignment first also indicates what secondary impairments are likely to develop, or are developing, because of the posture. Can his eyes only move in an upward gaze with this head position? Is the immobile position causing lack of self-initiated movement and, therefore, lack of development of good body awareness and body spatial awareness? Are joint contractures or areas of excessive range likely?

In children with hypotonia, the musculoskeletal system often tries to substitute for the lack of neuromuscular control. The child tries to use the integrity of joint structures and areas of muscle tightness to hold herself upright because she cannot use the neuromuscular control to do so. Specifically, she has trouble using patterns of cocontraction and sustained muscle activity. This often is the reason children with hypotonia assume the alignment they do. We often describe children with hypotonia as children who "hang on their joints," "fix themselves in a position," and "get stuck." In general, the therapist's job is to teach the child to replace dysfunctional musculoskeletal stability with control from muscle activity as much as possible. Then the child can do something functionally that she probably would not be able to learn to do given the way she is learning to move.

In children with moderate to severe involvement, begin working on the alignment and control in the head and trunk for a particular functional skill, choosing the skill based on the child's abilities, his age, the family's needs, and the future environment the child will function in. When working on the alignment and control of the head and trunk, two hands often are not enough, and equipment is required to help. A good place to begin is in the child's adaptive seating or in adaptive seating designed for his high chair. Ensure that no muscle group that needs to work is in an overlengthened position. If his head hangs forward with the rest of the spine rounded, the extensor muscles are in an overlengthened position. Align the child's head for him on top of a well-aligned trunk and proper base of support, then use visual, auditory, and proprioceptive input to help him hold his head where it is placed. This alignment asks him for an isometric contraction in his cervical and upper thoracic extensors.

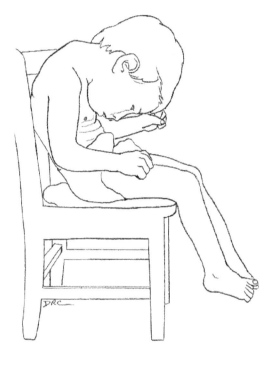

Figure 3.24 This 4-year-old boy shows severe over-stretching of his cervical and thoracic extensor muscles. His upper body weight is loaded onto his diaphragm, which compromises respiration in addition to the compromise in respiration caused by his elevated ribcage.

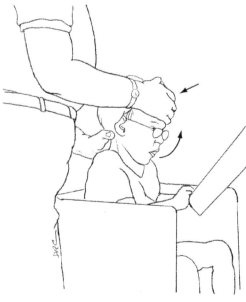

Figure 3.25 Here is one method that may be used to lift and place a child's head in alignment over an extended spine. The web space of one hand holds the child's occiput—be sure to contact and cradle the occiput with the entire web space of the hand for the child's comfort. The other hand is placed on the forehead, taking care not to cover the child's eyes. Both hands lift the child's head. The hand on the occiput can continue to give traction upward if the cervical extensors are tight and/or sustaining muscle activity too much. The hand on the forehead provides slight pressure toward the hand on the occiput; this directs the force necessary to give the child a chin tuck position of the head.

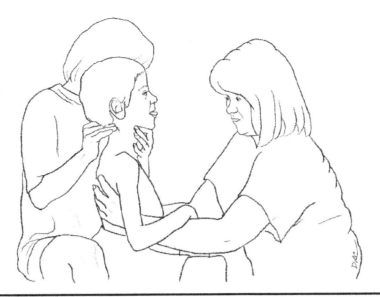

Figure 3.26 This 9-year-old's occupational and speech therapists facilitate alignment of his head and trunk carefully. The therapist in front of him holds his posterior-lateral ribcage, then brings her hands toward herself while at the same time pushing down against the seat he sits on. The therapist behind him holds his occiput and the base of his tongue to align his head over his spine and to ensure that his tongue is not retracted. They engage him visually to facilitate activation of postural muscles so that he can assist head control.

Use repetitive joint approximation through well-aligned joints (close-packed position) to help facilitate isometric holding, rarely using it through the top of the head. It is difficult to align the head perfectly with the cervical spine in good alignment. Rather, using joint approximation through the thoracic and lumbar spine works well to facilitate activity in the trunk for a more active base of support for the child's head to work from. As the child takes over holding her own head (her head doesn't feel so heavy when she takes over), check to see if she can begin to hold her head with decreasing support. Let go enough so that she can take the weight of her own head, but keep your hands very close so that her head does not fall forward or backward if she cannot take over. This enables her to practice head control in more functional alignment, yet gives her limited range through which she has to work, preventing her from overlengthening muscle groups. Continue to repeat proprioceptive, visual, and auditory cues if they help her hold up her head. This sensory information assists postural control and makes correct head alignment meaningful. She can see, hear, and perhaps touch a toy or a face that she sees and hears. She can feel a new body position and work to learn it. This may take some time—the new position may feel so different or frightening that she resists it or is otherwise unsure of it. If she is gently shown, though, that she can see a face or play with a toy that she likes, she may be convinced with time that the new posture is one that she wants.

Notice that the illustrations show the child in a sitting position. Prone is a very difficult position in which to work on head control (see Appendix A). Children with poor head control are more successful when in sitting or standing. In addition to the benefits of alignment, visual orientation, and less work against gravity in these positions, arousal/attention is better than in prone or supine.

In treating children with moderate to severe involvement in their head and trunk control, it helps to work with small ranges of weight shifting, involving the child as actively as possible, through the entire trunk. Placing and keeping the child in a small degree of rotation of the spine while the spine is extended helps the child stay more active and can assist beginning head control much better than staying in straight flexion/extension planes. Perhaps this is because the child cannot fall into gravity as well as when he is in the sagittal plane. It also may have to do with length-tension relationships of postural muscles: the deep extensors of the spine and the abdominal obliques are rotators of the spine. This also may be because rotation is a good place to facilitate cocontraction as the flexors and extensors must work in synergy to hold the rotated position. It also is a place where the child is less likely to hold his breath and is a good place to lengthen the intercostal muscles. The answer may involve all of these factors and perhaps a few more.

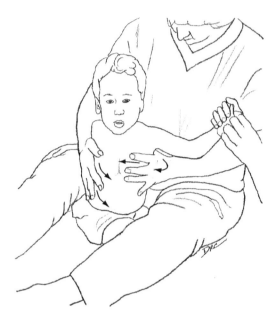

Figure 3.27 This 2½-year-old has severe hypotonia along with athetosis and some ability to stiffen his limbs with voluntary effort. His head is usually dropped forward onto his chest. He holds his head erect on his own when his therapist extends and rotates his thoracic spine.

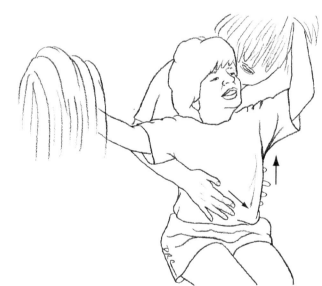

Figure 3.28 This 9-year-old is practicing her cheerleading. Her therapist is assisting her to take more weight on the left hip as the child lifts the left arm into the air. The therapist does this first by supporting the external abdominal obliques and left side of ribcage, and then exerts a diagonal force from the hand on the obilques toward the left hip *before* using her hand to help lift and spread the ribs.

When working on the head and trunk postural control in the child, it is important to remember that the reason for treatment is to gain function. You may be working toward the function of being able to look at toys, books, or people while she is seated fully supported in her adaptive chair. This requires addressing separating eye movements from head movements (see General Treatment Strategies in Chapter 6). You also may be working to get her to hold her head up long enough to take food offered to her on a spoon while seated in the same way. Maybe the goal is an assisted standing transfer, and this is where therapists must begin. Whatever the goal, work on the function once the child is actively assisting some part of the posture or movement.

In a child who can hold his head erect much of the time and sit on the floor independently when placed, but cannot get into sitting or standing, cannot feed himself with a spoon, and only vocalizes a limited number of brief sounds, the therapist is likely to work very hard on the trunk throughout the treatment session. The occupational therapist will use some of the strategies of trunk rotation and will add movement in and out of sitting with upper extremity weight bearing, decreasing physical support as needed, then returning to erect sitting to free the arms for spoon feeding. The speech-language pathologist may work in and out of active, assisted rotation with spinal extension for prolonged vocalizations as the ribcage becomes more mobile and the trunk more active. The physical therapist is likely to work much longer in weight shifting for some movement transition, such as getting in and out of sitting. All three therapists, however, are likely to need to work hard on gaining more active trunk control in this child at the beginning of the treatment sessions prior to working on the specific skill.

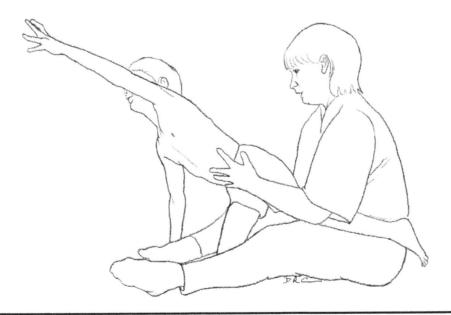

Figure 3.29 The therapist works with the child on active trunk extension with rotation. This may help facilitate postural extension for erect sitting. Here, the therapist supports his lower extremities in a disassociated position to help him assume a rotated position in the trunk. She also supports his lower extremities in a narrow base of support so that he can rotate his trunk as he is assisted to shift weight over his right leg. Her hand on his anterior trunk helps bring his ribcage down from its elevated position. Reaching overhead helps him actively lengthen the latissimus dorsi and intercostal muscles.

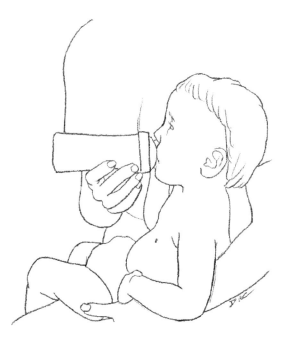

Figure 3.30 This 16-month-old is supported by her mother in more trunk extension with hip flexion than she began her therapy session with. The therapist treated her trunk, facilitating thoracic extension with rotation. This was followed by feeding the child her bottle, facilitating lip closure while progressively aligning her head in less cervical extension. As a home program, the therapist shows the mother how to support her child well in thoracic extension before giving her the bottle.

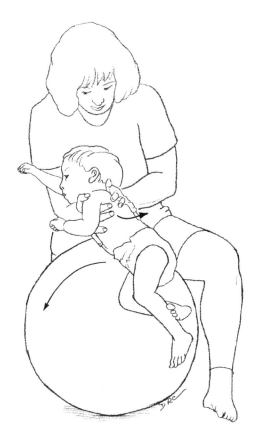

Figure 3.31 The therapist facilitates active trunk rotation as she assists this child to move between prone and supine on the therapy ball. The therapist moves the ball underneath the child in the opposite direction that the child moves. This ensures that the child stays on top of the ball. The ball's movement also assists the child to move more easily than if he were on a flat surface.

With a child who is ready for more graded control, look at narrowing the base of support in whatever posture you are working. Work to gain active trunk movement in all three planes so that the child can begin to decrease her base of support on her own. (Remember that one of the reasons that the child maintains a wide base of support is because of an inactive trunk.)

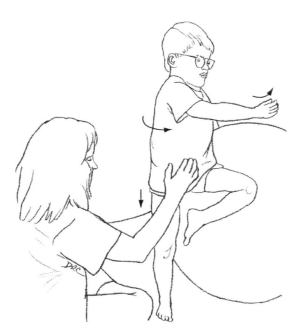

Figure 3.32 The therapist helps this 6-year-old stand supported on one foot while the ball supports some of his weight. One of the therapist's hands is on the child's abdominal oblique muscle group. As she moves the ball back and forth, she can slightly rotate the child's trunk to help him stay more active.

While in the more narrow base of support, continue to facilitate sustained holding of muscles and graded control of muscles around joints in ever more complex synergies. The synergies you choose to work on should depend entirely on the goal for treatment for that day. For example, if the goal is that the child puts on his own sock while sitting on a small chair or bench, then you may need to emphasize the ability to shift weight and hold with the abdominal obliques while the trunk stays relatively extended, because lifting the foot to hold it in the air and put a sock on usually requires shifting the weight back within the base of support. Shifting the weight back requires control of lower trunk flexion, usually with some small degree of rotation. You may need to work on the ability to hold the leg in the air for a short time using primarily the flexors of the hip and knee with the hip in external rotation. The child also could place the foot on the opposite knee after lifting it. The child may need to work on active plantar flexion of the foot, which makes it easier to put on a sock.

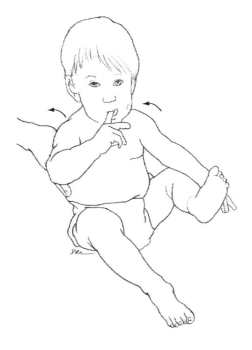

Figure 3.33 The therapist facilitates trunk extension, then tilts the child toward the back of his base of support *while maintaining the thoracic extension* to activate the abdominal muscles. He now is able to lift his foot so that he can assist with putting on a sock.

Children With Hypotonia

If the goal were that the child be able to produce a word beginning or ending with a bilabial sound, a speech pathologist may work on active head and trunk control as a base of support for the jaw to work from. Work to narrow the width of the legs in the position in which the child sits in order to enable the possibility of working the trunk more actively. Focus on keeping the trunk in a position of extension, but tilting the child back slightly to increase the likelihood that the postural flexors become more active in supporting the head and trunk. This often facilitates mouth closing. In addition, direct facilatory tapping to the facial musculature may increase the activity of the lips and cheeks. Ask the child to bite to increase jaw gradation or chew to increase tongue movements while in this posture. Some activities for oral feeders can include holding a cereal loop between the lips to facilitate activity in the lips and cup or straw drinking. For non-oral feeders, activities such as bubble blowing or giving kisses could facilitate lip activity. Ask the child to say the word or words that require the bilabial sound indicated in the goal, perhaps alternating with the activity that encourages active lip closure. Words that end in the bilabial sound are often the easiest to accomplish first (for example, u*p* and mo*m*).

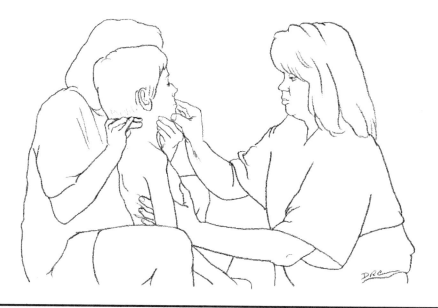

Figure 3.34 This child's occupational and speech therapists help him hold trunk extension alignment prior to tilting him back slightly. His OT helps him hold his head aligned over his extended trunk. His speech therapist holds the base of his ribcage to assist thoracic extension. She then facilitates lip closure. She also keeps him visually engaged to facilitate proper head position.

For the physical therapist, the goal may be that a child who walks learns to step up stairs without a handrail. She currently cannot do this because she does not support weight long enough on one leg to lift the other onto the step; she does not know how to shift weight to do so. She also does not have the strength in the lower extremities to lift her body weight. The physical therapist first might work on the weight shift necessary to lift and place a foot. Again, in this example, control of lower trunk flexion with slight rotation is required because the weight transfer is onto one foot with much of the weight on the heel. However, the trunk and supporting lower extremity stay in extension with this weight shift, and the trunk extensors and hip, knee, and ankle extensors also have to be active. This is a difficult and often frightening weight shift for a child with poor neuromuscular control. The physical therapist must work on placing the foot on the step in such a way that the base of support is not too wide, because if it is, the child cannot transfer weight onto this leg to rise. Also, if it is too wide, the hip abductors are at a poor length-tension relationship to stabilize the hip. The child must switch to using trunk extension with rotation control to rise onto the step. She also must work on the strength of the hip, knee, and ankle extensors necessary to lift her body weight.

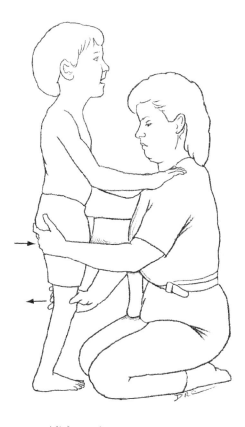

Figure 3.35 This child has been assisted to place his foot on his therapist's leg. The therapist has taken care that his hips are in neutral to slight external rotation and that they are adducted to neutral. She helps him with hip and knee extension on the stance leg. She also can shift his weight slightly in the sagittal plane to help him place more or less weight on his heel. When his weight is on his heel, he needs to contract his dorsiflexors, quadriceps femoris, and abdominal muscles to keep him upright.

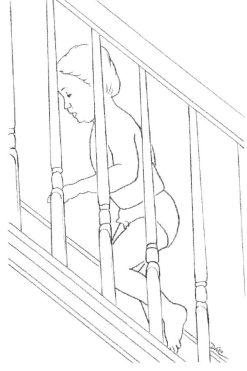

Figure 3.36 In climbing up a stair step, the trunk is extended as the child's weight moves over the forward foot. The trunk starts in a position of extension with rotation, and then derotates as the child brings the other foot to the same step.

Finally, in considering even more complex skills, the child with hypotonia often needs work on quick, reciprocal movements that require change in direction. These are skills that eventually could be addressed with children who progress well on more basic skills or those who are more mildly involved. The therapist may work on respiratory, muscular, and cardiovascular endurance. For example, if the goal is to be able to run in a soccer game for a set number of minutes without having to sit out on the sidelines, the difficulty often is that the child holds his breath while running. The child does this to generate trunk stability—the breath holding generates internal stability to substitute for postural muscle stability. Of course this does not enable the child to run for very long. The physical therapist must help him coordinate breathing with running, first by working on increasing trunk postural activity while in standing and walking, and then by adding running to the stability gained in the trunk. The child has to keep talking as he runs to let the therapist know he is breathing!

The speech pathologist may have a goal that the child be able to talk more rapidly and in longer sentences to enter conversations more easily. This requires controlled exhalation (in addition to many oral motor requirements) and quick initiation of voicing. The therapist may need to work on the alignment necessary for adequate intake during inhalation, followed by graded exhalation using abdominal obliques and intercostal muscles. To be sure the alignment supports adequate air exchange, the thoracic spine must be extended enough to enable ribcage mobility. The therapist may need to work on the child's ability to actively expand the ribcage while breathing and talking, using support of the abdominal and intercostal muscles while exhaling. Finally, add to this the ability to move around—that is, walk and talk at the same time.

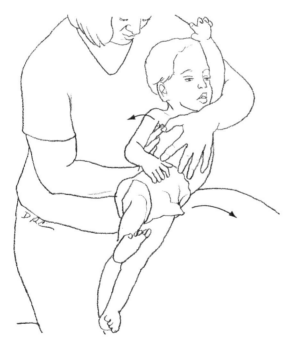

Figure 3.37a The therapist continues the work seen in Figure 3.31. She uses her left hand to spread the child's anterior chest open as her right hand moves down toward his pelvis to help bring his ribcage down from its elevated position. This helps elongate the intercostal muscles.

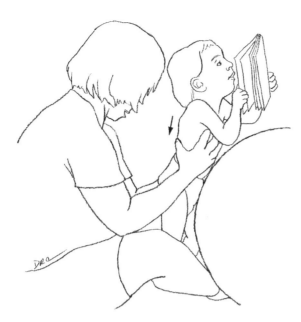

Figure 3.37b The therapist continues to elongate the intercostal muscles as she brings the child into a standing position. His center of mass is still forward in his base of support, and he is not yet as active as he needs to be throughout his entire trunk for standing control. This is evidenced by his use of excessive cervical extension to try to assist standing.

As the child's occupational therapist, you may have a goal for the child of being able to write in cursive script in a certain amount of time to complete a classroom assignment. The child may have difficulty orienting and holding the paper with one hand. With her writing hand, she holds the pencil with a grasp that relies little on the intrinsics of the hand. During writing, movement comes from the shoulder, with the wrist unmoving. The pencil presses too lightly even though her fingers grip it tightly. In treatment, you may decide that one of the problems is in interlimb coordination—the ability to make one limb use a different synergy of movement than the other. This may be the reason for the difficulty in holding the paper with one hand while the other writes. Work on more simple but relevant activities that require one hand to hold while the other moves. This requires an active trunk. You also may work on activities that promote use of active wrist movements with a stable shoulder in the hand that writes.

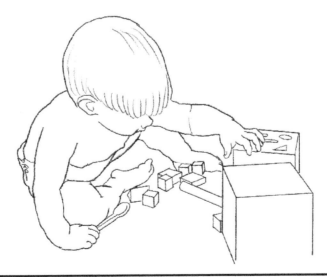

Figure 3.38a This child leans on one hand while reaching with the other. Note that he is controlling his trunk in all three planes. His right hip also is actively pushing down against the floor as is his left foot. In treatment, use active assisted trunk rotation prior to weight bearing with one arm.

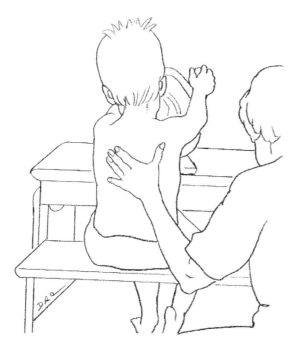

Figure 3.38b The therapist assists this child to play with a toy that requires one hand to hold the toy while the other pulls a lever. She assists him to sustain thoracic extension during this activity. The combination of active thoracic extension when the arms are at about 90° elevation is difficult. This can be true for people with normal central nervous system control too; it is easy to slump into thoracic flexion as we work at a desk.

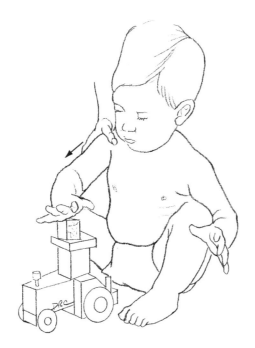

Figure 3.39 The therapist assists this baby to actively release a toy. The baby is just beginning active release, so has not developed initiation of this movement with wrist extension yet. The therapist supports the baby's shoulder, assisting shoulder stabilizer muscles (the rotator cuff) to give the proximal stability for distal control.

Now, look at two children with hypotonia and follow a treatment sequence toward a functional goal. The first is an 8-year-old girl who can sit in an adaptive wheelchair and classroom chair. Both chairs have custom-made seating with contoured seat and back, a head support system, lateral trunk supports, anterior straps to help hold her trunk upright, a seat belt, foot rests with straps to hold her feet against them, and a detachable tray. The child is able to look and follow horizontally with her eyes about 30° to either side of midline while fully supported in these chairs. Without the support of her seating systems, her head drops forward and she is unable to lift it in any position.

She lifts her eyes into an upward gaze while seated in her chairs to indicate *yes* and makes an "ahh" sound while she shakes her head slightly to indicate *no*. She is consistent and accurate with these responses. A speech pathologist will help her learn to shift her gaze to make requests for a food choice presented to her. Her mother wants her to communicate more than just *yes* and *no* responses, and the child already clearly has food preferences (she closes her mouth and/or tries to turn her head away from foods she does not want, or cries if food she wants is removed). A functional goal is that she can look at a food she wants or

wants more of. As therapist, you want her to learn that she requests a food or more of a food by looking at it, looking at whoever is feeding her, and looking at the food again. This requires that she learn to look down at her tray, look specifically to the left or right to indicate choice while looking down, and shift her gaze up to a face, and back down to the food.

You may begin treatment out of her seating systems, in order to facilitate more active trunk and head control. Taking her out of her seating offers an opportunity and creates a disadvantage. The opportunity is for her to further develop head and trunk control (by keeping her in her supportive seating she cannot do this). The disadvantage is that she is 8 years old and has developed very little control, so there are probably many impairments that contribute to her lack of control. You may choose to treat her on a large (39" diameter) therapy ball that enables you to place her on her stomach and also enables you to bring her into a nearly vertical position. This supports the child's trunk and thighs while also providing her the advantage of gravity assistance to actively hold up her head. You can support and stabilize her pelvis against the ball while facilitating thoracic extension and upper-extremity weight bearing.

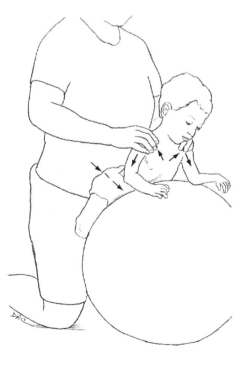

Figure 3.40 The therapist assists the child to hold his head erect while he looks down as he is supported in a near vertical position on a therapy ball. This is the position described for the 8-year-old girl with difficulty holding her head erect on pages 47–48. In this drawing, the child can hold his head upright as he is given support at his lower body and as his shoulder complex is brought down out of elevation and into more scapular adduction with thoracic extension. As he continues to become more active with cervical and upper thoracic postural control, the therapist will decrease his lower extremity base of support and facilitate lower trunk postural activity.

The alignment of the girl's trunk and hips along with the upright position helps her hold her head up for brief periods (5–10 seconds at a time). This is different from what she does in her seating systems because it involves much more upper trunk and cervical muscle activity.

As she is able to hold her head erect, play a game with her that involves looking straight ahead and slightly to one side. As she does this, support her mid- to lower trunk and pelvis while assisting her trunk to rotate ever so slightly in the direction she is looking.

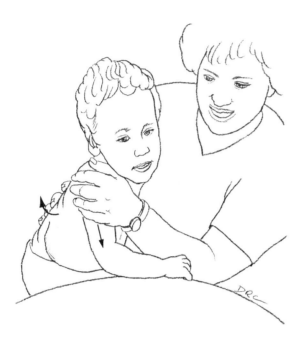

Figure 3.41   The therapist assists this child to extend and rotate his thoracic spine as described for the 8-year-old on pages 47–48. Active assistive thoracic extension with rotation is one of the best ways to facilitate postural control of the head.

Following this activity, seat the child in one of her chairs. You may have to determine how many of her straps and supports to use and how much to let her control her own posture (many straps and supports in seating systems can be loosened or removed temporarily).

Together, play a game in which the girl has to look at you, look at a toy or other object, and look at you again in order to be given the toy to play with or to have the toy activated for her. This also may be practiced with snack food.

Have the child's mother give you a food the child likes and one that she does not like so that the child learns to look at the one she likes. Give the girl a choice of two things to eat. She must look at you or at her mother, look at the food she likes, and look at the adult again to make the choice. By placing the food on

something on top of her tray that elevates it almost to eye level, the girl does not have to try to use as much downward gaze. You may need to reapply all of her straps and supports for this new and difficult functional activity.

As the child becomes consistent in this new motor task, slowly lower the food to tray level, which will require some movement of her head as well as more excursion of downward gaze. Her parents should practice this activity at home while the girl sits in her chair. Show her parents how to help her shift her gaze after finding the best way to support her in her chair. The seating system should support her so that her parents do not have to try to support her posture as well as get her to look where she needs to look. This may take some work in therapy sessions to figure out.

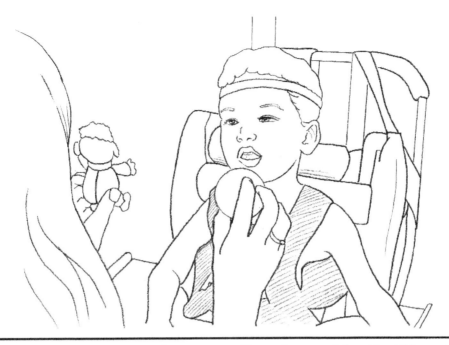

Figure 3.42 This child is seated as described for the 8-year-old on pages 47–48. The wheelchair is custom-made and includes a head support system. The therapist holds two toys at eye level for the child to choose from with eye gaze.

The active control that this child uses is the eye gaze and shift of the eyes from one toy to the other. Work on head and trunk postural control make use of eye movements much smoother for most children.

The second child is a 5-year-old who has mild hypotonia. He was born at 35 weeks gestation and had some primary respiratory impairments as an infant that resulted in asthma. He is able to walk, run, play outdoor games, talk, draw shapes with crayons, feed himself, and dress himself except for fastenings and shoe tying. He has trouble keeping up with peers in his kindergarten class on the playground and cannot get on and off the swings by himself. He does not run as fast as his classmates. He cannot ride a two-wheel bicycle. He cannot cut with scissors and is slower than anyone else in his class in printing letters of the alphabet. People who don't know him well often find him difficult to understand. He occasionally drools when he is doing tabletop fine-motor activities.

For his physical therapy goal, he and his family have decided that he wants to play soccer on a YMCA team. He has begun practices with the team of 5-year-olds, but he and his family are worried because he tires easily and cannot seem to run as fast as the other children.

He holds his breath for difficult motor activities, including running and scissor cutting, but maintains even respiration for motor skills that he has mastered. Breath holding often is done to generate internal trunk stability when the postural muscles may not work adequately to support posture or movement for the task. When he runs down a soccer field, he probably holds his breath a good deal of the time, contributing to his early fatigue. He has difficulty changing direction as he runs and difficulty orienting his foot to the ball (even more so than other 5-year-olds who also are learning ball management skills). This is because of his difficulty in quick initiation of movement with a new synergy, as well as his difficulty using trunk postural muscles to generate trunk rotation. He can move his trunk and hips in all three planes if given several seconds delay in initiating the movement or in switching to a different synergy to change direction of movement. He can perform many skills when speed is not the critical issue.

You work to increase his ability to initiate and change synergies of movement more quickly. Start with familiar movements that require power from lower extremity extension, but no trunk rotation or direction change (e.g., jumping with both feet). Increase the speed of repetition of jumping with auditory and visual cues. For example, many children organize initiation and repetition of movement more quickly and automatically when given an auditory rhythm to follow. This can be as simple as counting or singing a tune with words or a repetitive syllable, with a definite starting and stopping place to the rhythm. Use visual constraints to help organize the child's movement. For example, have the child jump in a square marked on the floor. These treatment ideas often work well for children who have impairments of higher levels of control and coordination. They also work in teaching new skills to children who are developing normally.

As the child initiates movements more quickly, use several ways to increase the complexity. Eventually, you will need to combine all of these strategies to help the boy run more efficiently and to orient his foot more to the ball. First, allow him to continue practicing the jumping or a well-mastered skill while he talks. Then increase the speed as he talks so that he is coordinating breathing with the movement when he speaks on controlled exhalation. Next, add direction change to the jumping activity or a similar activity. You first might ask for direction change with whole body movement, such as repetitive jumping, then introduce increasingly more difficult direction change with trunk and/or hip rotation. Or you first might ask for a slower speed such as walking and kicking, then ask for running and kicking with a ball coming from different angles each time. Finally, you might have him practice a simulated game of soccer, where he runs and controls the ball. Communicate with the boy's soccer coach to tell the coach what works best and to ask for suggestions about having the child practice talking and running at the same time.

The child's mother and teacher also want the boy to learn to cut with scissors in occupational therapy. The child holds the scissors with his right hand and is able to hold the paper with his left hand. While sitting at a small table and chair, he attempts to chop at the paper with the scissors. However, because of poor alignment of his entire body, he cannot take more than an occasional, uncontrolled jab at the paper. This is caused by weakness in the postural extensors of the trunk and compensatory postures to substitute for the stability given by these postural muscles. He also has poor ability to sustain wrist extension and radial deviation of both wrists when needed, and poor interlimb coordination, so that one arm has difficulty using a different set of muscles and producing different movements than the other arm. The child uses a slightly rounded thoracic posture with elevated and abducted scapulae, an elevated shoulder complex, slight shoulder internal rotation, excessive elbow flexion with slightly pronated forearms, and the use of wrist flexion with ulnar deviation and no variability to this wrist posture, a skill necessary for reorienting the scissors. His head also is in excessive upper cervical extension as the task becomes more challenging, which makes it hard for him to use eye movements free of head movements for constant visual contact with the paper he is cutting.

You may begin treatment to facilitate the use of the deep trunk extensors for postural holding of the trunk in more extension. You may choose to work in sitting or standing. In either case, you must align the thoracic spine carefully in more extension and shift the boy's center of mass toward the front of his base of support to elicit an extension response actively. This may be accomplished with a slight degree of thoracic rotation so that the child is biased to use the deeper extensor muscles of the trunk.

Add upper-extremity weight bearing, shifting body weight over the arm as much as the child can actively hold with the rotator cuff and triceps. It is critical to combine thoracic extension and rotation with this weight bearing to facilitate scapular adduction. You should ensure that this shoulder is not excessively elevated and is in neutral to slight external rotation. Your hand may cover the shoulder to support it the way the rotator cuff muscles do. You may decrease support as the child actively takes over. You and the child could play a game that requires him to shift over the arm and back again. Ensure that the elbow is extended but not hyperextended and that the wrist is extended and slightly radially deviated. The boy's

hand may be supported in weight bearing by a toy that cups the hand the way the arches should.

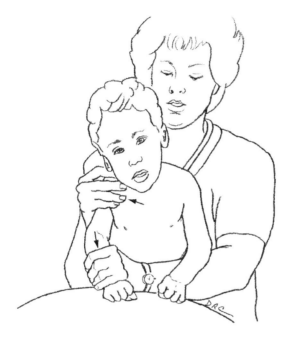

Figure 3.43   The therapist supports the child's shoulder over the rotator cuff muscles and assists elbow and wrist extension with weight bearing.

Continue the reaching game so that one arm is weight bearing and the other is reaching (interlimb coordination and upper extremity dissociation), remembering that sustained thoracic extension with rotation will be the best postural activity for this limb control. Then move to a tabletop activity that enables you to assist shoulder position and forearm stability while the child is actively working on tasks in the hand with wrist extension and radial deviation. The child could begin with toys that only require grasp and release, toys that require graded grasp and release to use, and scissors that require grasp with graded opening and closing and a variable wrist position. You may ask the child to work on cutting with some part of his arms supported on the tabletop rather than trying to use the scissors while holding the paper in the air.

The posture gained in sustained work of thoracic extension is likely to greatly assist head position needed for freer eye movements. However, with the better head position, the child may not know automatically how to use

his eyes to lead head movements or to sustain downward gaze when needed. If this is a problem, work with the eye movements once the head posture improves with more postural extension. To facilitate downward gaze, tilt the child back toward the back of his base of support, making sure that the trunk stays as extended as possible. This often facilitates a chin tuck. This can be done while the child is well seated in his chair by lifting the front legs of the chair and placing them on small blocks of wood. You could ask the boy to look at you or at a toy while looking straight ahead and then to begin shifting his eyes slightly down he is tilted back. You could ask him to begin to shift his gaze from one target to another when his posture is more active and sustained. For example, he could look from one picture in a book to another with the book held directly in front of him. Then you could ask him to look at a bottle of bubble soap on the tabletop in front of him (downward gaze), and then to look straight ahead at the bubble wand before he blows the bubble. Then you could return to the tabletop activities described.

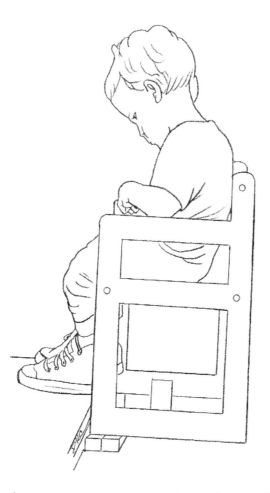

Figure 3.44 This child is sitting in a chair that has been slightly tilted back with blocks under the front legs of the chair. Care is taken to ensure that his pelvis is not posteriorly tilted and that his thoracic spine is extended. He then is able to look down.

For his classroom program, you could show the boy's teacher how to support his wrist as he practices cutting with paper. Give the teacher a different pair of scissors that open and close more easily to try with the child.

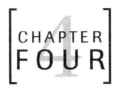

Children With Hypertonia

Pathophysiology

Children with hypertonic cerebral palsy represent the largest group of children who have CP (Albright, Cervi, & Singletary, 1991; Parker, et al., 1993; van den Berg-Emons, et al., 1996). This group includes children with quadriplegia, diplegia, and hemiplegia. *Quadriplegia* is used to describe a child who shows involvement of the entire body. These children are often moderately to severely involved. *Diplegia* represents a distribution of involvement of the lower body greater than that of the upper body. *Hemiplegia* refers to involvement on one side of the body with a presumed unilateral lesion of the CNS.

Hypertonia is used in this text instead of spasticity. Although hypertonia and spasticity are used by many authors interchangeably, others distinguish between the terms. Spasticity is a positive sign of CNS dysfunction. The most classic definition of spasticity used in the literature is by J. W. Lance (Lin, Brown, & Brotherstone, 1994): "In both cerebral and spinal spasticity, the stretch reflex responses obtainable from extensor and flexor muscle groups of the upper and lower limbs increase in the velocity of stretch. Therefore, the reflex component of the increased tone might be measured in terms of the threshold velocity required to evoke reflex activity and the slope of the EMG-velocity relationship." *Spasticity* therefore is defined as a reflexive, sensory initiated type of abnormal tone. *Hypertonia* is excessive resistance to movement, arising from both reflexive and non-reflexive elements (Carey & Burghardt, 1993).

In looking at children with cerebral palsy, the impairments involve more than the positive sign of spasticity. They also include negative signs such as loss of normal agonist-antagonist relationships (excessive cocontraction), loss of the ability to terminate movement at will (excessive sustained muscle activity), loss of muscle extensibility, and loss of some sensory/perceptual abilities. In addition, there are nonreflexive components of increased muscle tone such as changes in the properties of muscular and connective tissues that contribute to resistance to active and passive movement, making the limbs of children with CP more stiff (Boiteau, Malouin, & Richards, 1995; Brown, 1993).

Therefore, *hypertonia* is a broader, more inclusive term to describe children with CP who are too stiff. *Stiffness* is a relationship of force and length and is defined in muscle as a ratio of the change in force to the change in length. At a joint, the stiffness is the ratio of change in torque to the change in angle. Forces are all forces acting on the muscle or joint, both internal and external. Therefore, hypertonia is a term that enables various possibilities for an increase in resistance to movement—spasticity, excessive cocontraction, muscle and connective tissue property changes, and abnormally sustained muscle activity. Hypertonia also is a term that is more relevant to the many impairments that need to be evaluated and treated in children with this type of CP.

Finally, and equally as important, of the impairments that could be influenced in therapy, spasticity (reflexive, velocity-dependent stretch) may not be what is changed. The Bobaths used to say that we changed spasticity or hypertonus when we treated children (Bobath & Bobath, 1964; Bobath, K., 1971). Certainly we change something—it is clinically observable that children who are too stiff can decrease this stiffness when treated. But what is it that is really changed? Many clinicians now speculate that it is not spasticity, but the negative signs of the lesion, that is, the amount of cocontraction the child generates and sustains, the ability to initiate and terminate movement more easily, the use of more functional postural and movement synergies, and the extensibility of muscle and connective tissues.

Children with spasticity probably have damage to the corticospinal (pyramidal) tracts that descend from the motor cortex (Sutherland, 1984). There can be a variety of lesions that ultimately result in this damage. Because many lesions result in spasticity, it is reasonable to think that the variety of lesions also result in many different negative signs of CNS dysfunction in addition to the positive sign of spasticity.

Children with quadriplegia may suffer cerebral hypoxia that causes global involvement of the CNS (Gage, 1991). This can be seen on neuroimaging as cavities that communicate with the lateral ventricles, multiple cystic lesions in the white matter, diffuse cortical atrophy, and hydrocephalus (Kuban & Leviton, 1994). Because the damage is diffuse, these children also often have impairments from seizure activity and cognitive impairments.

Children with diplegia often are born prematurely and are prone to lesions of the periventricular white matter of the lateral side of the lateral ventricles, which more selectively influence optical function and lower body movement (Crawford & Hobbs, 1994).

Children with hemiplegia often show unilateral structural damage or maldevelopment in the CNS when born full term, have injury to the middle cerebral artery, or show subdural or intradural bleeding seen with resultant periventricular white matter damage when born prematurely (Kuban & Leviton, 1994; Wiklund & Uvebrant, 1991). Children with hemiplegia have a high incidence of seizure development as they grow. Many also have profound learning impairments (Goodman & Yude, 1996; Wiklund & Uvebrant, 1991).

However, it often is not possible to predict the distribution of the type of cerebral palsy or the extent of the disability based on the size or location of the lesion (Olney & Wright 1994). For example, on magnetic resonance imaging (MRI), or other diagnostic testing, there appears to be a continuum between diplegia and hemiplegia when the location and extent of the lesion is described.

Impairments

Neuromuscular system

Reflexive tone

In children with hypertonia, there may be abnormal reflexive tone. Spasticity can be present with abnormally increased velocity-dependent stretch reflexes.

Difficulties with muscle contraction

Children with hypertonia have difficulty controlling initiation and termination of movement. They show excessive sustained muscle contractions, which they have difficulty terminating. These sustained contractions conceivably can be in patterns of cocontraction or in patterns of more reciprocal inhibition where the agonist sustains firing while the antagonist is not firing at all. Clinically, it is easy to see that children with hypertonia have difficulty turning off muscle contractions. Because of this, many clinicians develop treatment techniques specifically to help solve this problem. Rapid joint oscillatory movements imposed on the child, manual vibration, and sustained traction are some of the techniques therapists use to help children terminate muscle activity or grade termination of muscle activity.

Children with hypertonia move slowly or have paucity of movement. A partial explanation of this is that such children have problems initiating, sustaining, and terminating movement. These problems can be primary problems of lack of the CNS to recruit or to turn off activity. They also can be secondary impairments when the sustained activity is a voluntary effort to control joints. For example, many children with hypertonic CP have trouble initiating muscle activity. There often are two areas that the therapist must attend to when trying to help the child learn to initiate—the alignment or starting position from which the child is trying to initiate activity and the ability of the child to terminate activity in the antagonist so that he can initiate it in the agonist. Often, the therapist is at least partially successful in helping the child both terminate unwanted antagonist activity and initiate the desired agonist activity by carefully aligning joints and body segments prior to the effort to move. This is the use of good kinesiological principles.

This careful attention to alignment has always been a core part of the NDT approach to treatment. It is one reason why therapists who use the NDT philosophy find that hands-on treatment for at least part of each session often is necessary.

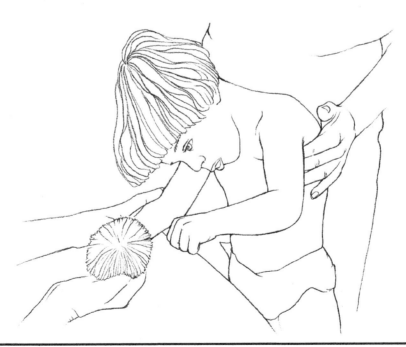

Figure 4.1 This 3-year-old is trying to reach for a toy with her left hand. Her thoracic spine is actively held in flexion with her shoulder internally rotated, elbow flexed, forearm pronated, and wrist flexed with ulnar deviation. She is unable to initiate wrist extension in reach.

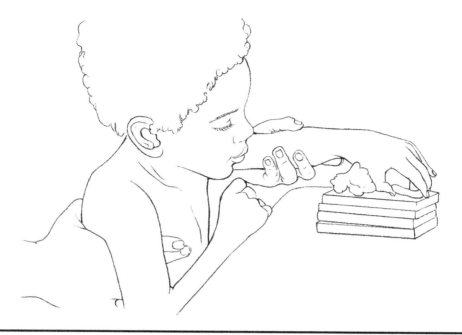

Figure 4.2 In treatment, this child's therapist uses techniques to first align his thoracic spine in more extension and shoulder in less internal rotation. His wrist will be aligned in slight extension and radial deviation with his forearm in a more neutral position. With support by the therapist or by another weight-bearing surface, this new alignment prepares him to terminate wrist and hand flexor activity. The therapist also may need to help him terminate flexor activity with additional treatment techniques. If needed, the therapist then can facilitate wrist extension for reach or the child may be able to do it on his own.

Grading agonist/antagonist activity

In children with hypertonia, there is an abnormal ability to grade between cocontraction and reciprocal inhibition. There often is excessive cocontraction in voluntary efforts. This increases neuromuscular stiffness in the limbs and sometimes in the trunks of children with hypertonic CP. In some instances, this increase in stiffness is seen as an immature or disordered ability of use of the agonist-antagonist relationship, and therefore, would be a primary impairment (Berger, Quintern, & Dietz, 1982; Brogren, Hadders-Algra, & Forssberg, 1996; Dietz & Berger, 1995; Leonard, Hirschfeld, & Forssberg, 1991; Nashner, Shumway-Cook, & Marin, 1983). In other instances, children with hypertonia may use increased stiffness as a compensatory strategy to control posture and prevent unwanted or uncontrolled movement in other areas of the body (Nashner, et al., 1983; Brogren, et al., 1996). Because excessive cocontraction in children with hypertonia may come from a variety of sources—a primary impairment, an immature response to postural perturbations, or compensatory holding against other dysfunctional movements—the results of treatment aimed at reducing unwanted cocontraction during movement vary.

In addition to these possibilities for overuse of cocontraction, the distribution of the ability to use and sustain cocontraction in children with hypertonia varies. This further complicates the picture. Many children with quadriplegia or more severe diplegia often are described as having a hypotonic trunk with hypertonic limbs. How can this be? Clinically, it is clear that the therapist sees very stiff limbs and a floppy, inactive trunk in these children. There are several possibilities that may explain this phenomenon:

- Once again, the idea that postural muscles react differently than mover muscles to any lesion may provide some explanation. If the therapist observes closely, the *hypotonic* trunk often shows inactivity in the postural muscles with holding of the mover muscles—the pectorals, scapular elevators, and latissimus dorsi.

- Children with hypertonia may not only have a problem with excessive cocontraction, but have a problem grading its use. This may mean that they are capable of only an all-or-nothing approach—either excessive cocontraction or nothing at all. And for whatever reason, the limbs often are able to take the *all* approach, whereas the trunk can take only the *nothing* approach.

- If the cocontraction is compensatory, as it often is seen clinically, then there is some reason why the limbs are able to generate more muscle activity than the trunk. It is for this reason that in this text the problems of children who use excessive cocontraction are regarded as *hypertonic* instead of *spastic*. Many children can generate compensatory cocontraction to stiffen their limbs when they lack control of their trunk. Children with spasticity can do it, but so can many children with hypotonia, athetosis, and ataxia. Many times children who are ataxic are misdiagnosed as spastic because they learn how to hold so well with limb cocontraction to avoid any change in their center of mass while moving. Their limbs are indeed very stiff, but many of them are not at all spastic. Compensatory cocontraction is a secondary impairment.

It is tempting to think that much of the change seen in children with hypertonia during treatment is because so many use cocontraction to stiffen themselves when they do not have the graded control needed in the trunk or limbs to execute skilled movement. The changes seen by Mrs. Bobath, who believed that she changed or reduced spasticity, may really have been changes in the voluntary cocontraction that many children are capable of—from children with spasticity to children with hypotonia. Remember that children and adults who have normal neuromuscular systems also use excessive cocontraction in new or unskilled situations.

Any new therapist has learned some techniques to *relax* children or *reduce tone*. But relaxing children often reduces arousal/attention (e.g., the use of slow movement; a darkened, quiet room; rocking). Rather than relaxation, therapists must evaluate more specifically the impairments they want to change. If stiffness due to sustained cocontraction in non-functional synergies is the biggest problem, then treatment must focus on changing this while focusing arousal/attention on a functional task. If therapists are truly able to help children grade the use of cocontraction, develop more skilled agonist-antagonist relationships, and change the alignment from which they initiate their patterns of cocontraction, then the words *relax* and *reduce tone* are not appropriate.

Limited synergies used to produce posture and movement

The child with hypertonia may show several problems in use of postural and movement synergies. This is an area that probably has been researched more than any other neuromuscular impairment in children with CP. Nashner et al. (1983) found that the postural synergies used by children with hemiplegia were abnormal as the children tried to control postural sway on a platform. Temporal order was reversed in the legs on the hemiplegic side—the children showed a proximal to distal ordering of firing of muscles rather than the normal distal to proximal ordering. This ordering of muscle firing tends to destabilize rather than stabilize posture. The forces of the contractions also were quite variable. This study also showed that there was increased coactivation of antagonists with the agonists when attempting to correct postural sway, lending support for abnormal use of cocontraction. One of the conclusions of the study was that the lesions that cause cerebral palsy may result in primary impairments of altered CNS programs that impose inappropriate temporal and spatial structure on synergies.

Therapists would benefit from a study investigating whether the timing and ordering of these basic synergies changed when the child's alignment changed. Researchers could test the child as he or she typically stands, then record the timing and ordering of muscle synergies. Would these synergies be different if the child were then aligned differently? Would they be different with therapeutic practice? And if they were different, what effect would this have on function? Therapists know clinically that alignment, weight shift capabilities (movement of the center of mass in relation to the base of support or anticipated base of support), available passive range of motion, and sensory cues can influence the synergies that children use to initiate and execute movement. However, therapists must see research results to know more specifically what happens. As Lee (1984) points out, neuromotor synergies overlap with biomechanical, cognitive, and task-oriented factors.

If clinicians are correct in believing that alignment, range of motion, sensory feedback and feedforward, and weight shifting prior to initiating movement affects and changes the use of synergies, then the problem of synergy use in children with hypertonia also can have components of secondary impairments, as well as the primary impairment of disordered timing and ordering of programs suggested by Nashner et al. (1983). These secondary impairments are certainly more easily changed in a therapeutic session. Perhaps therapists do influence CNS changes by more correct practice, but they also can immediately influence alignment, weight shifting, and sensory conditions provided those sensory conditions can be processed and used.

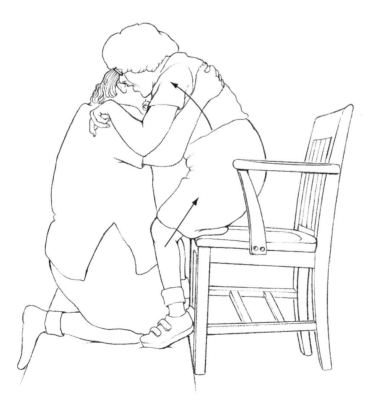

Figure 4.3 This 16-year-old quickly initiates activity in her medial hamstrings and hip adductors, which pulls her into hip extension with adduction/internal rotation, pushing her center of mass back. She also initiates with plantar flexion of the ankle in the shortened range with her heels off of the floor as she is helped to stand. She therefore has difficulty moving her center of mass forward far enough over her feet prior to initiating extension to rise to stand. She has to compensate with overuse of her upper body to pull herself onto her feet.

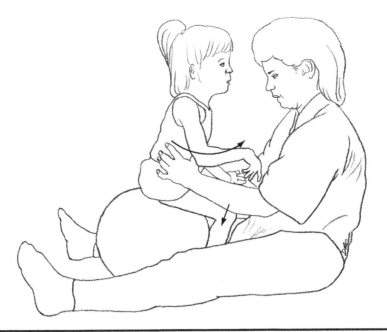

Figure 4.4 This 4-year-old's therapist is making sure that the child is sitting with trunk extension and hip flexion prior to helping her take pressure through her feet. Her therapist may spend time giving deep tactile pressure and/or proprioceptive input to her feet and through her ankle joints if her impairments include a high threshold to perceiving sensory information. With attention to this alignment and preparation of the new base of support the child needs for standing, the therapist facilitates the possibility of the use of lower extremity joints using active extension to rise to stand as her center of mass moves forward and up over her feet.

Sensory/Perceptual systems

The child with hypertonia may have both primary and secondary impairments in vision. Children with hypertonia frequently show primary impairments in the visual system that include ocular motor and cortical processing problems (Cioni, Fazzi, Ipata, Canapicchi, & van Hof-van Duin, 1996; Ito, et al., 1996). Because of strabismus, higher integrative disorders such as quick localization, smooth pursuit of moving objects, and depth perception often are affected. Visual field losses are common, especially in hemiplegia. Errors of refraction and accommodation result in difficulties learning fine motor skills and accomplishing educational tasks (Duckman, 1979, 1984, 1987). Duckman outlines remediation efforts that therapists can use in children with cerebral palsy for some of these problems.

Children with hypertonia also may show secondary visual impairments. As with other children with any type of cerebral palsy, children with hypertonia often use upward gaze (eye extension) to assist postural extension. When performed from the slightly asymmetrical head position frequently seen in children with hypertonia, the child may learn to use the eyes almost exclusively in one of the upper quadrants. Over time, with disuse, it is possible that much of the normal visual fields are lost.

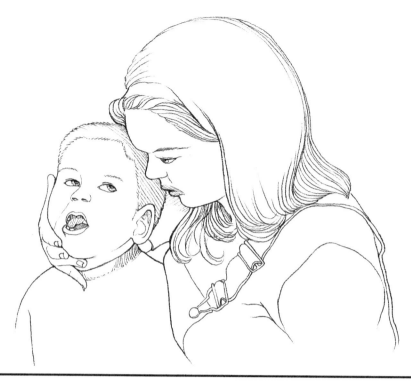

Figure 4.5 This 4-year-old is vocalizing. He pushes out his air during exhalation with lower extremity and trunk extension. He also uses eye extension (upward gaze) as part of the overall extension synergy to vocalize. Because this eye extension is initiated with his neck in asymmetrical extension, the eyes tend to deviate to one quadrant.

Children with hypertonia are thought to use abnormal sensory feedback when trying to grade grip and anticipate closure of the hand during manipulation tasks (Eliasson, Gordon, & Forssberg, 1992). This, as well as impaired neuromuscular skills, results in abnormal grip forces, abnormal timing of muscle activity, and a poor ability to anticipate shaping of the hand to objects. Other researchers have looked at possible impairments of vestibular function and kinesthetic senses.

Therapists must better understand the role of sensory information in motor performance in children with hypertonia. Are all of the impairments primary, or are there secondary impairments that result from lack of movement or movement from abnormal postures? Are the thresholds of sensory feedback loops (the critical excitatory input required to fire an action potential of the nerve cell) abnormal, or are there central processing problems that make error detection through sensory systems impossible? Clinically, many children with hypertonia seem to show abnormal thresholds as opposed to central processing problems. This is because providing children organized tactile, proprioceptive, and vestibular information as they move often helps them learn new functional tasks. Thresholds may be the bigger problem because in some children, especially those with hemiplegia, there may be areas of hyposensitivity and areas of hypersensitivity, especially to tactile information.

In children with hypotonia there is a great sensitivity to sound, even more than in children with other types of cerebral palsy. Loud, sudden, or unexpected sounds often elicit an exaggerated motor response. With experience of these reactions, children and their families try to avoid or are constantly aware of the possibility of encountering sounds that produce such responses. This indicates a possible impairment in threshold of receiving auditory information. Likewise, many children with hypertonia have a sensitivity to and fear of change of position, either imposed on them or self-produced. This may be a specific vestibular impairment or a problem caused by sensory sensitivity in combination with range of motion (ROM) limitations and neuromuscular impairments (that is, delayed initiation of movement, poor synergy selection to support or protect the body, or excessive cocontraction that prevents support or protective responses).

Musculoskeletal system

Clearly, children with hypertonia develop joint contractures and muscle shortness from the neuromuscular impairments of excessive cocontraction and excessive sustained muscle activity (Tardieu, de la Tour, Bret, & Tardieu, 1982; Tardieu, Tardieu, Colbeau-Justin, & Lespargot, 1982). Thus, this loss of range of motion is a secondary impairment. The muscles that tend to shorten are more superficial muscles, two-joint muscles, and muscles that were originally shortened at birth. Many muscles fall into all three of these categories and tend to be the ones for which gaining range is extremely difficult. Examples of the three categories can be found in Appendix C.

In addition to the muscles that typically shorten because of these conditions, therapists also may want to consider other issues that ultimately affect joint position. Because a child with hypertonia uses excessive, sustained muscle activity around a joint, the joint tends to rest in a position favorable to the muscle with the largest cross-sectional area. Therefore, one reason the forearm tends to pronate, in addition to the infant retention of short pronators, may be that the pronators are thick and deep compared to the pull of the supinators. In the ankle, the foot often rests in a plantar-flexed position. It is true that the gastrocnemious may be overactive and/or shortened, but it also is true that the gastrocnemious is much larger in cross-sectional area than the muscles that dorsiflex the ankle. Therapists who have seen the ankle pull hard into dorsiflexion after Achilles tendon lengthening may suspect that the dorsiflexors were always overactive, but were simply overpowered by the larger plantar flexors until lengthened.

Children with hypertonia also show secondary impairments in the skeletal system. Because children are affected not only by neuromuscular influences, gravity, and nutrition, but also by growth, the bones and joints have several sources for altered growth and structural changes. Again, children with hypertonia present with the primary impairments of excessive cocontraction and excessive sustained muscle activity. When imposed on a poorly aligned skeletal system that is growing, the potential for altered and restricted development is great. Remember that constant compression on growing bone restricts its growth (LeVeau & Bernhardt, 1984).

Bony changes in the spine and ribcage

In the spine and ribcage, there are several common structural changes that develop over time. The ribcage tends to stay elevated with lack of effective lower trunk activity to anchor it to the pelvis. There are two common shapes to the ribcage.

- The ribcage is barrel shaped, presumably due to tightness and/or overactivity of the trunk muscles, including the intercostals, erector spinae, diaphragm, and rectus abdominus; this might be viewed as a problem of excessive muscle activity. In addition, the thoracic spine is kyphotic to a certain degree.

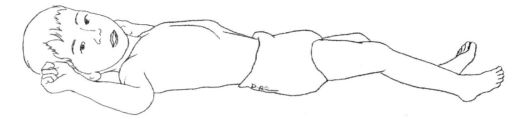

Figure 4.6 This 4-year-old with spastic athetosis lies supine. Note the increased anterior-posterior diameter of his chest. This indicates his constant effort in respiration. His intercostal muscles are prob- ably short and possibly overactive, as are his superfi- cial trunk muscles. The shape of his ribcage is seen in other diagnoses where the person fights for air (e.g., emphysema).

- In children who have more difficulty activating trunk muscles, the ribcage often looks similar to that of children with hypotonia—a flattened anterior- posterior diameter, flaring of the distal ribcage, an elevated ribcage with hori- zontally positioned ribs, and a rounded thoracic spine.

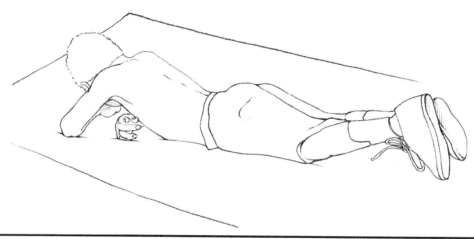

Figure 4.7 This 4-year-old sustains muscle activity in the trunk and limbs with superficial muscles that span more than one joint. He has difficulty activating postural muscles. In the trunk, he has difficulty acti- vating the deep postural trunk extensors, the inter- costals, and the abdominal muscles. As a result, his ribcage has remained in the elevated position typical- ly seen in much younger children. He has poor abdominal support of the distal ribcage so that there is lateral flaring of the ribs. With poor muscular sup- port of the ribcage and with the pull of gravity, the anterior-posterior depth of his ribcage is decreased. His upper thoracic spine is pulled into flexion as his arms pull him along the floor, which reinforces the elevation of his shoulder complex and ribcage.

With time, either of these shapes become more structural, limiting respiratory capaci- ty, trunk movements, and balance.

Another common structural deformity that develops in many children with hyperto- nia is scoliosis. Estimates of this secondary impairment are as high as 25–76% in an institutionalized population (Cassidy, Craig, Perry, Karlin, & Goldberg, 1994). Curves usually are most progressive in children who have more severe involvement and are non-ambulatory. Curves in children with quadriplegia are often long, C- shaped thoracolumbar curves (Aronsson, Stokes, Ronchetti, & Labelle, 1994). These curves can be progressive even after skeletal maturity, well into at least the third decade of life (Thometz & Simon, 1988). Problems with pain, skin breakdown, respiratory problems, and functional deterioration are commonly reported (Brashear & Raney, 1978; Cassidy, et al., 1994; Staheli, 1992).

The exact causes of scoliosis in children with cerebral palsy are unknown. The likelihood is that there are multiple primary and secondary impairments that contribute to its formation, including:

- imbalance of trunk muscle activity that is either an imbalance of superficial versus deeper postural muscles activity, of flexion and extension activity, of right side verses left side, or a combination of any of these;

- a retention of kyphosis in the entire spine or in the thoracic spine. Kyphosis (flexion or forward bending) is an open-packed position of the facet joints; therefore the spine is structurally more unstable and may be more vulnerable to influences by any abnormal internal or external forces; and

- poor sensory and perceptual skills from somatosensory, visual, and/or vestibular systems, tending to result in feedback that causes the child to assume persistent asymmetrical postures and movements.

Clinically, young children with hypertonia who are less active with postural trunk muscles and who are more severely involved (usually quadriplegic) first develop a long, C-shaped thoracolumbar curve with all of their active and passive lateral movement taking place about the thoracolumbar junction.

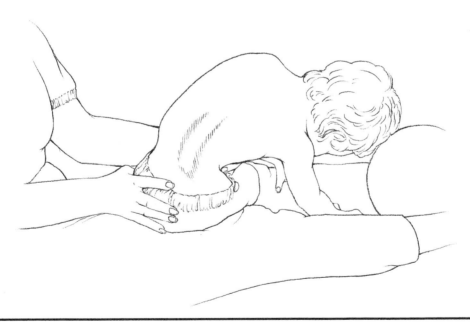

Figure 4.8 This 2½-year-old has very poor ability to use any postural holding in his trunk, although he can activate and sustain some muscle groups in his limbs. Without external support of his trunk, he collapses with a C-shaped lateral curve of his spine. With time and habitual positioning this way, a structural as well as a functional scoliosis can develop.

Sometimes this curve changes to a more S-shaped curve, and sometimes it tends to remain C-shaped. The typical movements the child makes undoubtedly have an influence on this development.

Children with hemiplegia and children with hip dislocation more frequently develop lumbar scoliosis, perhaps because of a greater influence of pelvic asymmetry when sitting or standing.

In preparing to manage scoliosis, especially while it is still functional as opposed to structural, the therapist must be aware of all the possible influences of multiple systems that could cause it. In addition, the therapist must remember how the scoliosis begins to change the shape of the spine and ribcage and influence muscle pull.

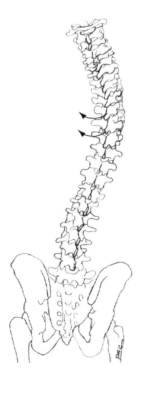

Figure 4.9a The thoracic spine on this skeleton shows scoliosis with relative extension. It represents what is typically thought of as the biomechanics of scoliosis—the vertebrae rotate so that the spinous processes move toward the concavity of the scoliosis. This curve with the concavity on the left would produce a rib hump posteriorly on the right. This may be seen in children with cerebral palsy who have scoliosis.

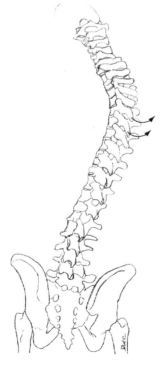

Figure 4.9b The thoracic spine in this skeleton is in flexion with scoliosis. Note that the vertebral bodies rotate to the side of the concavity. The rib hump would be on the left posteriorly. In some children with severe trunk flexion and scoliosis, this may be the biomechanics of their curve. This can be confusing to the clinician who expects the rib hump to be opposite the concavity of the curve as is typically seen and discussed in textbooks.

Changes in other bones and joints

Changes in other bones and joints in addition to those of the ribcage and spine are common in children with hypertonia.

Hip

A subluxed or dislocated hip is one of the most researched and well-known impairments that develops over time (Cornell, 1995; Laplaza & Root, 1994).

There are many influences on the development of the hip in children with hypertonia that result in a subluxed or dislocated hip. Because of this, many researchers do not agree on the primary or most influential causes of hip problems. Likely impairments that influence the eventual outcome of subluxed or dislocated hips in children with hypertonia are:

- The retention of the structural shape of the infant acetabulum and femur (Cornell, 1995; Laplaza & Root, 1994; Pope, Bueff, & DeLuca, 1994). The infant acetabulum is shallow, and therefore, offers poor stability to the hip joint. In the infant developing normally, this instability is protected by muscle tightness around the hip. The infant femur shows a neck-shaft angle of about 140° with femoral anteversion of about 40° (Cornell, 1995). These angles change with growth and muscle pull in the infant developing normally so that the neck-shaft angle is about 125° in the adult with about 14° of femoral anteversion.

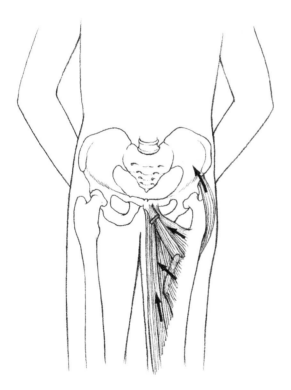

Figure 4.10 The gluteus medius (hip abductor) and the hip adductor group pull the femoral head in toward the acetabulum when they contract in hip extension. This deepens the acetabulum in a growing child. It also makes the neck-shaft angle more acute as the adductors gently shape the femur over time so that the shaft of the femur shapes into an adducted position.

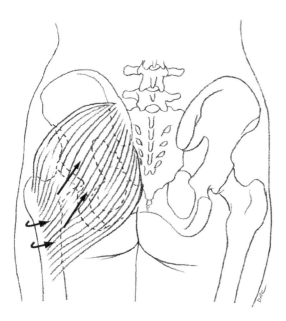

Figure 4.11 The normal pull of the active gluteus maximus extends and externally rotates the hip joint. The ligaments over the anterior surface of the cartilaginous femoral head also reshape the femur into less anteversion when the hip is extended as they are stretched taut. You can see by its insertion on the posterior proximal femur that as the gluteus maximus pulls, it may shape the growing bone, decreasing the internal twisting of the long axis (decreasing the degree of femoral anteversion). Many children with cerebral palsy do not effectively activate the gluteus maximus or activate it only with overpowering antagonistic activity of the hip flexors and internal rotators. Therefore, the normal activity of the gluteus maximus in changing bony structure with growth is diminished or absent and the anterior ligaments of the hip do not push against the femoral head because the hip is not extended.

- In children with hypertonic CP, the muscle pull on the developing hip is markedly different than in children developing without CP. Children with hypertonia show an imbalance of muscle activity, usually with strong pull of the hip flexors, adductors, and internal rotators (medial hamstrings). This may influence development of the hip bony structure, as well as cause subluxation and dislocation of the hip over time (Cornell, 1995; Pope, et al., 1994).

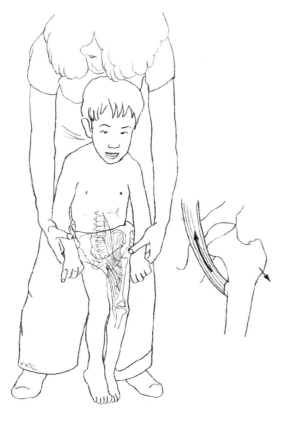

Figure 4.12 This child stands with his therapist's assistance. His hips pull strongly into slight flexion and adduction. As these muscles pull relatively unopposed, they tend to exert most force on the medial side of the femur, thereby pulling the head of the femur away from the acetabulum laterally. Hip subluxation or dislocation results.

Knee

The knee changes that result from the primary impairments in children with hypertonia are well documented. The knee often flexes in response to abnormal biomechanics of movement, especially gait, with a resulting flexion contracture (Gage, 1991; Perry, Antonelli, & Ford, 1975; Sutherland & Cooper, 1978). The knee also often ends up with a flexion contracture because of sustained cocontraction around the knee joint. Occasionally, the knee hyperextends due to hip and ankle pathomechanics during gait (Gage, 1991; Simon, et al., 1978). In order to successfully treat problems of the knee in movement, the therapist must understand the abnormal mechanics at all trunk and lower extremity joints.

Ankle and Foot

The ankle and foot changes that result from the primary impairments in children with hypertonia are the subject of entire books as well as research articles (Carmick, 1995a; Carmick, 1995b; Hainsworth, Harrison, Sheldon, & Roussounis, 1997; Mossberg, Linton, & Friske, 1990; Perry, Hoffer, Giovan, Antonelli, & Greenberg, 1974; Radtka, Skinner, Dixon, & Johanson, 1997; Rosenthal, 1984). In addition, many continuing education courses for therapists address this specific problem.

The common secondary impairments in the ankle and foot in children with hypertonia are:

- **Equinus (plantar flexed ankle).** This most likely starts as a muscle imbalance, with the dynamic function of the gastrocnemius and its large cross-sectional area influencing the ankle to assume the position of plantar flexion. Plantar flexion also can be a compensation for shortened hip and knee flexors or leg length discrepancy. In these cases, the plantar flexed ankle is merely a compensation to make a shorter leg reach the floor.

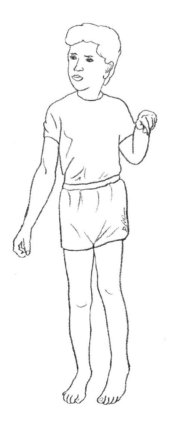

Figure 4.13 Plantar flexion may result as the large gastrocsoleus exerts more force than its smaller antagonists in the presence of abnormal reflexive and voluntary muscle activity. Plantar flexion also may be a way that this child with hemiplegia who elevates his pelvis on the left reaches the floor.

- Pronation or supination of the foot when weight bearing. This is a much more complex phenomenon, causing changes in all three planes of movement. It is likely due to a combination of muscle imbalances and abnormal forces in weight bearing.

Long Bones

Finally, there is evidence that many long bones in children with hypertonia grow abnormally (Lin & Henderson, 1996). Many children with CP show decreased bone density, increased incidences of fractures, and small stature. There are multiple factors influencing these findings. Excessive, sustained muscle activity tends to retard rather than promote bone growth. Medications and poor nutritional status can be other factors as can decreased use and atrophy of muscles that normally pull on a growing bone to stimulate growth.

Muscle Develoment

The child with hypertonia shows definite problems in strength development. This can be a primary impairment of the inability to generate muscle forces. There also are suggestions that the normal distribution of fast and slow twitch motor units are altered in some children with CP as either a primary or secondary impairment (Castle, et al., 1979). Clinically, therapists see the lack of strength development in certain ranges due to abnormal alignment to generate effective muscle pull, excessive activity of the antagonist, contractures and bony changes, abnormal external forces on poorly aligned joints, and disuse of the muscle in any functional synergy. However, certain muscles show great strength in some ranges in which they commonly work. Therefore, the issue is not whether or not a particular muscle is strong or weak, but where in the range is the muscle strong or weak, with what other muscle activity is the muscle able to produce force (that is, what synergies can the muscle work in and what synergies does it not work in), and how much of the range is available for the child to use.

For example, in many children with hypertonia, the biceps brachii are active in a synergy of shoulder complex elevation, shoulder joint extension with internal rotation, and forearm pronation. They tend to be used in a range of some flexion to more flexion, but not as good initiators of flexion from full extension. Although the biceps are biomechanically the primary forearm supinator, in children with hypertonia they are rarely effective supinators because of the shoulder position of strong internal rotation and the tightness/overactivity of the forearm pronators and long finger flexors.

In ambulatory children with diplegia, the quadriceps femoris often is very strong and overdeveloped proximally as it tries to stabilize the knee against many forces that would flex it in gait. However, the patella tends to sit high (patella alta), with overstretching of the patellar tendon, making terminal knee extension impossible biomechanically, even if the child has the range and the ability to isolate and produce force with this muscle.

In the head and neck area, the tongue often is held in retraction with the spine in capital extension (head on atlas) and the lower cervical and upper thoracic spine in flexion. This overstretches the infrahyoid muscles responsible for fixation of the hyoid bone and for control of cervical flexion. These muscles may not develop strength and control because of poor alignment.

Respiratory system

Children with hypertonia show many changes in their ribcage and thoracic spine structure over time. Therefore, many of the impairments in the respiratory system are secondary impairments. As detailed on page 71–72 on musculoskeletal system impairments, the ribcage begins to take shape because of muscular action or lack of action. The ribcage is either barrel shaped with excessive, sustained superficial muscle activity or is flattened with distal rib flaring because of a lack of activity in any muscle group. The result is that respiration often is shallow with an immobile ribcage during inhalation and exhalation. In both instances, the ribcage also is elevated. Because the thoracic spine is more kyphotic than in the child developing normally, the expansion of the anterior portion of the chest is limited, further impairing the depth of respiration.

Children with hypertonia often hold their breath as they vocalize or verbalize, enabling only a small stream of air to escape. They also often perform many of their gross and fine motor movements with breath held. This is true especially if the trunk has any activity in the more superficial muscles. Breath holding is a compensatory effort to stabilize the trunk with internal pressure when the postural muscles of the trunk cannot perform this function. It enables the child to hold the trunk erect to execute a skilled movement in the rest of the body, although only for short periods of time as the child must eventually take a breath. The results are that the child speaks with a very strained voice, can speak only in short phrases, and can move only for short periods.

Coordinating breathing with movement and speech involves proper trunk alignment; smooth gradation of muscle contractions; sufficient movement in joints, muscle length, and proper bone structure; and the complex control of a variety of movement synergies. All or any combination of impairments in these requirements compromise respiration for movement and speech production. Respiration can also be compromised by primary impairments that cause the child to inadequately ventilate. All of these impairments can be very subtle in more mildly involved children. For example, the child only holds his breath when he runs, and therefore, does not have the endurance to play on the playground, or he cannot speak fast enough to enter conversations when several people are trying to talk at once.

Quadriplegia
Typical Posture and Movement Strategies
Head, neck, tongue, and eyes

The child with quadriplegia uses slight asymmetrical extension of the cervical spine to hold up the head as she lifts it from the typical infant position of asymmetry. However, because the child either begins to use excessive sustaining of muscle activity or cannot sustain muscle activity sufficiently (some children with quadriplegia will show one problem and some the other), head control and position begin to alter early from that of babies developing normally. It is not unusual for children who have hypertonia to show the same or similar problems as children with hypotonia in the head, neck, and trunk. (See Chapter 3 for a discussion of the implications of insufficient activity of cervical postural musculature.)

Children who develop excessive muscle activity in the cervical area learn to hold, and keep holding, this slightly asymmetrical head position, extending the head on the neck and the neck on the trunk. The child holds in this posture most of the time during any attempts at postural control, so that the posture is strengthened and becomes unopposed. The child often holds the head only to one side. Early asymmetrical extension is not abnormal, because babies developing without CP use it too, but it is the only movement the child with CP can make. Upward visual gaze, tongue retraction, and jaw extension are easy movements for this child to make in synergy with cervical extension.

The difference between the child with hypertonia who uses upward visual gaze, tongue retraction, and jaw extension and the child with hypotonia who does so are:

- The child with hypertonia uses more of a midrange position of the head in extension, having to hold it there with muscle activity. In contrast, the child with hypotonia can let it fall back or forward against the spine or chest. Therefore, although the child with hypertonia is likely to overstretch the infrahyoid muscles, he probably will not overstretch them as much as the child who rests the head against the spine.

- The child with hypertonia is more likely to actively hold with tongue retraction rather than gravity causing the tongue to fall back as is seen in the child with hypotonia. Along with this, the child with hypertonia often shows a bunching at the center of the tongue as the tongue muscles contract strongly in an attempt to stabilize the jaw and cervical spine by pushing against the palate.

- The child with hypertonia uses more active, sustained jaw opening (extension) than the child with hypotonia.

- The child with hypertonia often can hold the eyes with upward visual gaze (eye extension) in one upper quadrant only, because she often holds the head in extension to a preferred side.

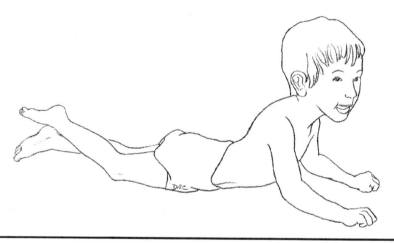

Figure 4.14a This child with spastic athetosis shows the slightly asymmetrically positioned head with cervical extension held actively and facial muscles active and tight.

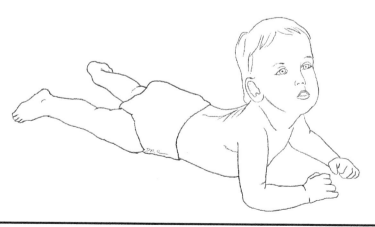

Figure 4.14b This child with hypotonia rests her head back on her spine once she has lifted it. Her facial muscles are underactive and her jaw drops open.

The child with hypertonia who controls the head with sustained, asymmetrical extension often develops tightness in these extensors and the loss of ROM in the upper cervical spine into flexion. Chin tuck and control of the eyes in all quadrants are difficult. Graded control of the jaw and separation of jaw from tongue movements are severely compromised.

Functionally, the child with hypertonia who excessively sustains extension in the cervical spine is unable to explore his environment visually. Depth perception does not develop because the eyes cannot work together in binocular vision. The child will have difficulty with feeding and sound production because of poor alignment of oral structures as well as the inability to terminate jaw and tongue postures to learn refined movements. The child is unable to control the cervical spine in any position except extension, thereby limiting range of motion and control for many functional skills, including orientation of the head to all sensory cues, even if the sensory systems do not have primary impairments.

A variety of disabilities can result. Speech often is poorly understood by those not intimately familiar with the child, and so communication via speech is ineffective with most people. The child may not be able to take all nutrition orally. Communication with the eyes, a very early form of reciprocal interaction with caretakers, may be impossible. Learning and exploring with the options of head and eye position become severely compromised, so that abilities such as reading, visually guided reaching, and locating objects or people in the environment are severely restricted.

The disabilities of an 8-month-old may include an inability to look at his mother when she bottle feeds him; to take baby cereal, fruits, and vegetables sufficiently to get adequate nutrition; and to visually locate toys when in prone or supine on the floor. A 4-year-old's disabilities may include the inability to look at a toy when he reaches for it while seated in his adaptive chair, a poor ability to chew food, and no understandable speech except a few words that his parents and teacher understand. A 10-year-old may have the disabilities of reading at only a first-grade level despite testing that shows his IQ to be in the low-normal range and an inability to get sufficient nutrition orally so that he has a gastrostomy tube in place for feedings.

Thoracic spine, ribcage, and upper extremities

Children with quadriplegia have a tremendous problem in learning to push against a surface with their upper extremities while lifting the head up. There may be several sources of the difficulty. Because the child is trying so hard to lift the head and recruits excessive extension, it may be impossible for her to use a more complex

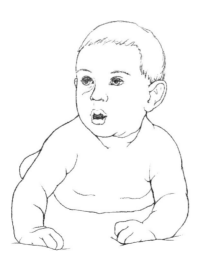

Figure 4.15 This 4-month-old baby lifts his head up as his arms push against the floor. He is developing the ability to lift and hold his head up with cervical and upper thoracic extension as well as a chin tuck. He pushes against the floor with his hands and forearms.

synergy of head lifting with extension in synergy with recruitment of the rotator cuff of the shoulders, the pectorals, and the scapular stabilizers. Instead, the head lifts and the arms lift, with shoulder extension and internal rotation, shoulder complex elevation, and usually minimal upper- to mid-thoracic extension. This may be an easier synergy to coordinate than the more functional one of cervical extension with shoulder flexion and horizontal adduction while stabilizing the scapulae.

If the child is using movements that are not helping him achieve function—that is, reach a toy, roll over, or stand at furniture with support—she may try harder. In trying harder, she recruits even more extension, and sustains that extension because this is what her central nervous system enables her to do. Instead of helping, though, the sustained extension only makes it more difficult to see anything in front of her, to use her voice effectively, or to balance in sitting or standing. The arms are used for postural control only rather than for stability in weight bearing or for reaching. When a child with quadriplegia can only use the arms to help lift the head, then reach, grasp, release, and manipulation become extremely difficult.

In addition to the difficulties with upper extremity function, the child with hypertonia who has a quadriplegic distribution shows difficulty developing extension control sufficiently and smoothly through the thoracic spine. At first, this may sound contradictory to the previous assertion that the child recruits too much extension. But look carefully at the child as he moves. What you usually see is that the child uses excessive and unopposed cervical extension with shoulder extension, but the shoulders and ribcage are elevated with the scapulae elevated and abducted. Because the shoulder complex is so elevated and the shoulders internally rotated (they are in this position at birth), it is impossible to use active extension throughout the thoracic spine. Try it yourself—don't forget to hold your shoulder complex very elevated and your shoulders very internally rotated. Then pull back with your arms into shoulder extension with your head also extended. You will see that the thoracic spine cannot extend much at all. The shoulder complex must let go of elevation, and begin to move toward shoulder external rotation for the thoracic spine to extend.

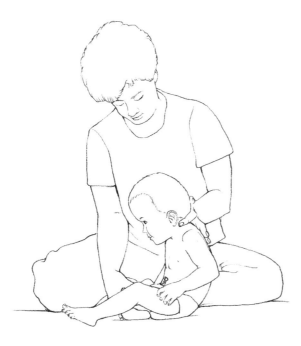

Figure 4.16 This 2-year-old with hypertonic quadriplegia sits with support only. Although he actively extends his cervical spine, shoulders, and hips (with the hamstrings, most likely), his thoracic spine is very rounded. It is tempting to think that because he pushes backward with extension that treatment should focus on flexion. However, this child needs assistance to actively extend his thoracic and lumbar spine with his hips in flexion. This is necessary to bring his center of mass forward over his legs for independent sitting.

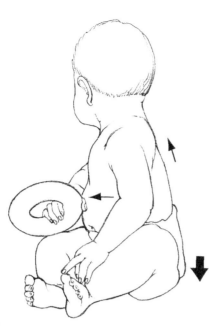

Figure 4.17 This 8-month-old sits with active trunk extension and activity of both hip flexors and extensors to control hip position. This enables him to shift his center of mass over his base of support. Note that his legs (his base of support) are in hip abduction and external rotation, whereas the child in Figure 4.16 has a more narrow base of support. In treatment work on all of these potential impairments: lack of a wider base of support, lack of active trunk extension, and lack of control around the hip joints.

Why does the child with quadriplegia stay in and use so much shoulder complex and ribcage elevation with shoulder internal rotation? One explanation is that the baby is born with the shoulder complex and ribcage in elevation and the shoulders internally rotated so that this is the initial position for all babies to begin movement. But babies developing normally soon change this initial position by controlling the head with extension, flexion, and rotation while pushing down with the arms against a surface (the crib, mother's shoulder). The more a baby can push into a surface, the more the pectorals and later the serratus anterior can work with the rotator cuff muscles. This changes the initial position of the shoulder complex to less elevation and less internal rotation as the shoulders move into flexion. The more the shoulders can start in a position of flexion, the better aligned the whole shoulder complex is for recruiting scapular stability and pectorals as horizontal adductors. This position enables alignment for effective, active thoracic extension throughout the entire thoracic spine. As mentioned in the review of normal development in Appendix A, there seems to be a strong relationship between the development of the ability to push against a surface with the arms and thoracic extension control.

So while the child with hypertonia who is involved throughout his body often sustains cervical and shoulder extension excessively, he does not develop thoracic extension actively. Therefore, when describing this child, the therapist should look carefully at where the child is able to produce and use extension. It is tempting to look quickly and see the movement into extension, concluding that treatment should focus exclusively on developing flexion control. This would not treat all of the alignment and control problems, however. You may find after careful evaluation (remember that not every child is going to fit this picture exactly), that you have to work hard on recruiting capital and cervical flexion and cervical rotation, pushing with the arms against a surface with less shoulder complex elevation and with shoulder flexion and external rotation. You also may find that you have to work very hard to recruit thoracic extension.

With exclusive use of cervical extension and shoulder extension with elevation and internal rotation, the pectorals shorten, as do the latissimus dorsi. Also with this proximal posturing, the elbow tends to flex as the biceps pull hard. The biceps are

Quadriplegia

not effective as forearm supinators (as they sometimes are in a similar proximal posturing after a stroke or head injury). This is probably because the shoulder is more internally rotated than in adults with acquired injuries, and internal rotation is a pronator assist. Also, in a baby and young child, the pronators of the forearm are not fully lengthened. Because of the short pronators, which are deep and thick in cross-sectional area, the forearm tends to pronate with elbow flexion. The hand follows with wrist flexion and ulnar deviation, finger flexion, and thumb flexion and adduction.

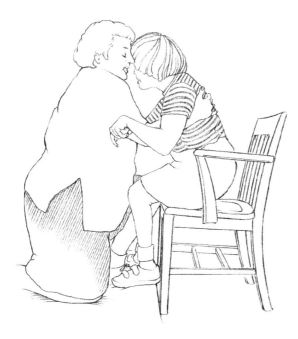

Figure 4.18 This teenager shows the positions described on page 83 of shoulder complex elevation, shoulder extension and internal rotation, elbow flexion with forearm pronation, and wrist flexion with ulnar deviation.

Functionally, the child with quadriplegia has an extremely difficult time using the upper extremities for any skill that requires reach, grasp, and release. The child often is so impaired that she can do nothing with the arms except use them as assists to head lifting. Others may be able to reach in a limited range, but usually are unable to do much with grasp or release. The harder they try, the more stiff they become in the effort. Breathing is compromised because the ribcage stays so elevated with the ribs positioned in a rigid structure. The continued thoracic kyphosis only places weight on the diaphragm when in sitting so that respiration is further impaired.

The disabilities that result are probably clear to the therapist. The child will have severe difficulties using the arms for any life role that involves anything more than limited range of reach and grasp. The child also cannot use graded respiratory control for speech, adequate ventilation for motor efforts, or for safe coordination with feeding. A 3-month-old may be unable to lift his head when placed in prone on the floor or held upright against his father's shoulder. He also never brings his hands together when held. A 3-year-old may have many disabilities, including the inability to play with any toy that requires grasp. She is capable only of pushing cars and balls using very limited ranges of movement. She can vocalize vowel sounds only. A 7-year-old can sit in a chair with support to his trunk and can grasp objects within a limited range, but cannot feed himself or assist in dressing. Because he tires easily, he does not have the endurance to participate in a full day of schoolwork that his teacher believes he is capable of academically.

Lower trunk

The child with quadriplegia often sustains muscle activity in muscles that are superficial, cross more than one joint, and/or were normally short at birth. In addition, the postural muscles of the trunk often are weak and inactive. Neuromuscular impairments, as well as poor alignment to begin and execute movement, contribute to the common picture therapists see in the lower trunk of children with quadriplegia.

The easiest synergy for this child often is lumbar extension with hip flexion, especially when in prone or supine positions. Perhaps this is because the child is trying to use so much extension in the upper body to achieve anti-gravity positions that lumbar extension becomes part of the effort. Lumbar extension is certainly easier biomechanically to achieve than thoracic extension, because the facet joints are in the sagittal plane and are made to enable the lumbar spine to work primarily in the sagittal plane. Lumbar extension does not require skilled control of the upper extremities to develop as does the thoracic spine. Also, the erector spinae cross many joints and are superficial muscles, so may be easy to recruit, producing lumbar extension more easily than thoracic extension. The deeper postural extensors such as the multifidous muscles and rotators that produce sustained, controlled extension and rotation may not be used much. Neither are the abdominal muscles, which are more postural in nature. The hip flexors are short at birth and are thick in cross-sectional area, so they may be easy muscles to recruit as well.

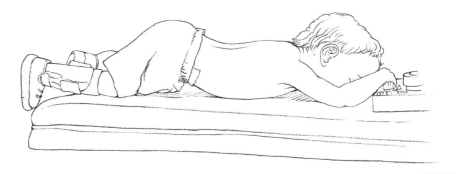

Figure 4.19 This child shows a typical position that a child with quadriplegia assumes—hip flexion with lumbar extension.

Another easy synergy for the child to recruit is sagittal plane flexion. The only muscle in the abdominal group that the child with quadriplegia seems to be able to recruit is the rectus abdominus, which has more mover than postural characteristics. This muscle works in the sagittal plane and might be biased by the flexion of the thoracic spine, which brings its origin closer to its insertion, especially when the child sits. This child uses active holding in trunk flexion with the pectorals and rectus abdominus as opposed to the passive drop into trunk flexion that the child with overall hypotonia is more likely to do. This also is aided by the strong contraction of the hip flexors and hamstrings, which pull the pelvis into a posterior tilt, seen especially in sitting.

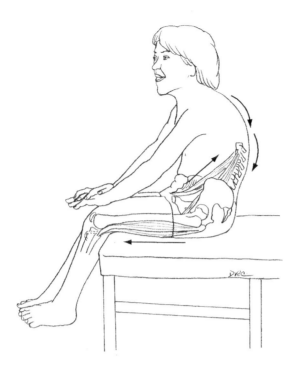

Figure 4.20 This teenager with quadriplegia tries to balance in sitting. She pulls hard with her pectoral muscles and rectus abdominus to bring her center of mass forward. This does not work, however, because her hamstrings pull hard too, causing her hips to extend, moving her pelvis into a posterior tilt. With her center of mass so far toward the back of her base of support, the contraction of her hip flexors lifts her thigh off of the mat and contributes to the posterior pelvic tilt.

As seen in the child with hypotonia, the child with hypertonia in a quadriplegic distribution may show a variable posture in the trunk when in different positions. The child with quadriplegia may show lumbar extension in prone and supine, but show flexion throughout the lumbar spine when sitting. Some children will switch synergies based on their position (prone versus sitting), whereas others become biased toward one synergy in all positions as certain muscle groups are overused and/or shortened.

Except for children with severe extension throughout the cervical and lumbar spine in all positions and with barrel chests from overactivity of the superficial muscles surrounding the ribcage, the child with hypertonic quadriplegia and the child with moderate to severe hypotonia can look remarkably similar in the trunk. Why is this? And what are the differences?

Consider the impairments that lead to the trunk posturing and lack of activity. Both children have abnormal neuromuscular control, which causes lack of activity in the postural muscles. Both have tightness in some of the superficial and two-joint muscles because of the lack of length shared by all infants and the limited variety of postures and movement they are able to perform—gravity acts on the few positions they can assume or are placed in. Children with hypertonia have more tightness in these muscles because of their ability to sustain holding with them. Therefore, they are likely to develop more contractures faster than children with hypotonia and are more likely to develop scoliosis and other ribcage deformities. Children with hypotonia, on the other hand, develop some contractures because of their poverty of movement and the effects of gravity on an inactive and immobile trunk.

In addition, neither child is able to develop sufficient control of thoracic extension, which involves a complex interaction of upper extremity control, a variety of synergies developing to control the upper trunk, and controlled lengthening of the muscles that were tight at birth. Therefore, it is not uncommon for children with any type of cerebral palsy to lack thoracic extension control.

Lack of abdominal use is another common problem seen in children with CP. The abdominal muscles are postural muscles that attach the ribcage to the pelvis anteriorly and are responsible for assisting in respiration, control of the lower trunk (and therefore the center of mass), and proximal stability for limb use. Because the muscles are primarily postural muscles, they lack activity both in children with hypertonia and hypotonia. In addition, the ribcage tends to stay elevated in both cases which frequently overlengthens the abdominal muscles.

Because the child with quadriplegia assumes a position of either lumbar extension or lumbar flexion without the control to grade movements between the two, he is biomechanically in a position of either open-packed facet joints when in flexion, or in the case of extension, close-packed joints (joint surfaces are the most congruent). Neither extreme gives the spine the alignment it needs to use thoracic rotation, an energy-conserving way to control the center of mass. As in the child with hypotonia, the child with quadriplegia often shows an inactive, unstable lower trunk that moves without control.

The child with quadriplegia has limitations in the role of providing stability for the center of mass. There is a further respiratory limitation that begins in the upper body—the abdominal muscles are poor support for controlled respiration and do not help anchor the ribcage toward the pelvis.

Disabilities that result are due to the limitations in center of mass control and in respiration. A 15-month-old cannot sit or stand because she does not have the postural control in the trunk to enable her to do so. She also cannot vocalize more than a few vowel sounds, as she does not stabilize with the abdominal muscles against the diaphragm during inhalation or control exhalation with graded termination of sustained abdominal contractions. She does not hold a cup yet or assist with upper extremity dressing by pushing her arms through sleeves because her lower trunk is not stable enough to enable her to use her arms for mobility—instead she tries to use her arms for posture, becoming stiffer as she sustains activity in many of the arm muscles.

A 6-year-old cannot sit unsupported in school and must sit in adaptive seating that substitutes for trunk control. This complex seating system, which has a seat belt, lateral hip and trunk supports, an abductor wedge, and a footplate, prevents him from learning how to get out of a chair himself because it has so many physical restraints. He can speak several words, but often is not heard in the noise of the classroom because he speaks softly. He therefore often remains passive about communicating his needs because past attempts often were ignored.

The pelvic girdle and lower extremities

It is here that the differences between the child with quadriplegia and the child with hypotonia are marked. The child with quadriplegia has many problems in function that start in this area of the body. Remember that the pelvis and legs are supposed to be used as a sufficient base of support for a variety of different positions. The hips also are needed for mobility and controlled movement for many functional skills. The child with quadriplegia has severe problems in all of these roles of the lower body. One of the biggest reasons is the sustained overactivity of many of the hip muscles, especially the flexors, adductors, and some of the internal rotators. Why these muscles and not their antagonists? Surely there are different lesions that can result in hypertonic quadriplegia from different insults to the CNS. Why do so many children with quadriplegia show the same problems of tightness in the flexors, adductors, and internal rotators of the hip and weakness or inactivity of the extensors, abductors, and external rotators?

There are no definitive answers and the explanations are likely to be derived from the interaction of many impairments. However, part of the likely answer is that the hip flexors, adductors, and the medial hamstrings (the internal rotators that seem to influence hip position the most in children with hypertonia) are muscles that are large in cross-sectional area compared to their antagonists—the gluteus maximus, medius, and the short external rotators. The flexor, adductor, and hamstring tendinous insertions are strong. The flexors are short at birth. The adductors and medial hamstrings include some two-joint muscles, whereas the gluteals and external rotators are one-joint muscles. The flexors, adductors, and medial hamstrings have longer lever arms. Therefore, it may be that the pathophysiology (the lesions) that causes quadriplegia would enable any of the hip muscles to be overactive, but because the flexors, adductors, and medial hamstrings have more characteristics that enable them to express this overactivity, they soon overpower their antagonists. Then, by pulling the hip into slight flexion, adduction, and internal rotation, the extensors, abductors, and external rotators may become overlengthened. They are in poor alignment to work effectively. Unopposed pull into flexion, adduction, and internal rotation sets the child up for early hip dislocation, which further compromises alignment, mobility, and development of the bony angles of the hip joint.

There are likely to be more comprehensive explanations for the biasing of hip flexion, adduction, and internal rotation in children with quadriplegia as more research is done. Regardless, children with hypertonic quadriplegia almost always show this hip posture. It results in a very narrow base of support, limited mobility, tightness and contracture of the overactive muscles, weakness and inactivity of the antagonists, early hip dislocation, and malformation of the hip joint.

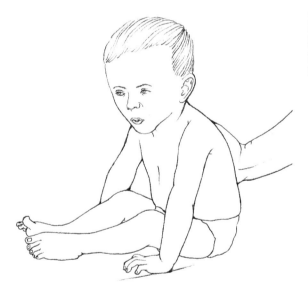

Figure 4.21a This child's narrow base of support is one of the contributing factors in his inability to sit independently.

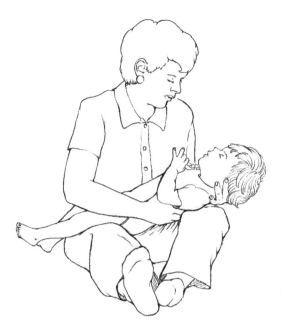

Figure 4.21b In supine or a reclined position, this child's hip flexion, adduction, and internal rotation provide little contact of his legs with the support surface. This will be one factor in making active transitional movements out of supine extremely difficult for him.

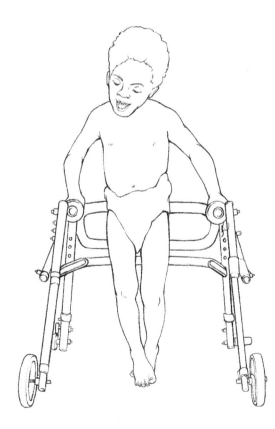

Figure 4.21c This child also has a very narrow base of support. He has many impairments that interfere with walking, and a narrow base of support makes shifting weight and balancing even more difficult. In treatment, a good place to start for work on many functional goals is to address alignment for a wider base of support in children with hypertonia.

Quadriplegia

The child with quadriplegia has two major areas of the body that work against upright control of posture—the inactivity of the trunk and a narrow, immobile base of support. At least the child with hypotonia could use a wide base of support to try to substitute for the inactive trunk, but the child with hypertonic quadriplegia does not have this option. As the child with quadriplegia feels insecure in a position she is placed in or begins to lose her balance, her only option is to increase the force of the contractions in muscles that already are overactive. Consequently, the child becomes *more spastic*. (This term is how many clinicians and writers have characterized this phenomenon, but it is unlikely that the reflexive abnormal tone changes as much as the voluntary stiffening.)

Functionally, the child is limited in the anti-gravity positions he can assume or maintain because of a narrow base of support, limited mobility, contractures, and bony malalignment.

Therapists can speculate about some of the ensuing disabilities. A 3-year-old is unable to sit because when she is placed in sitting her spine flexes into gravity, her hips are adducted and internally rotated so that there is very little surface area of her legs in contact with the chair, and her hips do not flex enough. This may seem to contradict what was said about hip position, but it does not. When the spine is flexed and the hamstrings are overactive, the center of mass moves backward. The hamstrings pull the hips into extension and internal rotation while flexing the knees. The hip flexors work hard at this point to try to hold on, but their action only tips the center of mass back even more.

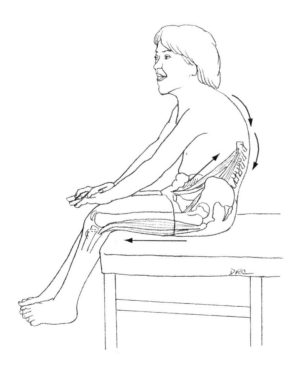

Figure 4.22 As this teenager with hypertonia sits, sustained activity in the hamstrings and hip flexors moves her center of mass toward the back of her base of support. If she tries to balance, she has to use flexion somewhere to bring her weight forward. She uses thoracic flexion and also may try to assist with the hip flexors. The problem is that when her hip flexors contract, her center of mass is too far back for them to effectively bring her trunk forward. Instead, as they cocontract with the hamstrings, the pelvis is tilted posteriorly, which continues to keep her center of mass toward the back of her base of support.

Chapter Four

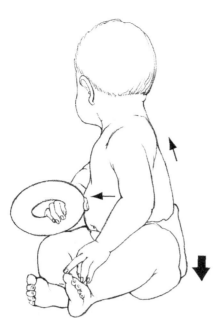

Figure 4.23 This 8-month-old sits with active thoracic extension and an active base of support. This includes active hip flexion and extension to make postural adjustments. His wide, lower-extremity base of support and his center of mass well within his base of support enable the hip flexors to move his trunk over relatively fixed legs. Because the psoas muscle attaches to the lumbar spine, the hip flexors can move the trunk over the legs when the center of mass is within an active base of support.

A 6-year-old cannot move from his position sitting on a bench because he is unable to shift his weight from the lower trunk and hips, rotate his spine, and use upper extremity support. He is stuck sitting where he is placed. A 16-year-old cannot independently transfer from her wheelchair to another chair for similar reasons. In addition, she has bony deformities and muscle contractures that make attaining a wider base of support impossible. She also cannot assist her mother in getting her out of bed in the morning.

General Treatment Strategies

Several approaches to starting treatment often are useful. After identifying the functional goals determined by the team of the family, child, and therapist, observe the child's posture in the positions and movements that he will need to make to accomplish the goal. Look first at the base of support. In children with hypertonic quadriplegia, the base of support often is a major obstacle to success in learning antigravity control and independent postures. First, work to get the best alignment and range of joint mobility possible to enable further work on active trunk control and movement of the limbs without so much stiffness. The following illustrations show some of the observations and work that can help prepare the child to hold antigravity postures and begin to move with control.

Another way to approach treatment, especially in children with very severe involvement who do not show head or trunk control in most postures and movements, is to look at the child's head and trunk stiffness and the alignment of segments of the spine. Often, children with hypertonic quadriplegia need assistance to increase the sustained control of postural muscles in the trunk while simultaneously decreasing sustained holding of superficial trunk muscles and limb muscles. This is why generalized relaxation techniques can be ineffective, as they relax everything, including the already inactive postural trunk muscles. Techniques that grade muscle activity more selectively, like manual vibration, which tends to inhibit sustained muscle activity, can be used on the overactive muscles, while joint approximation through well-aligned joints facilitates isometric holding around joints that need activity. When joint approximation is used through well-aligned joints, it does not usually increase unwanted stiffness. Nor does using localized manual vibration *relax* the whole body, but rather it helps the child terminate or grade muscle activity.

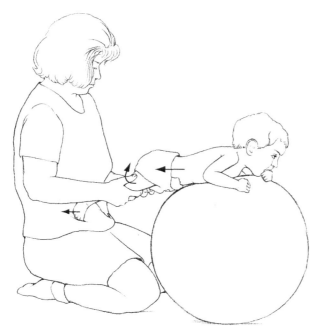

Figure 4.24   This therapist prepares the child's lower extremity alignment for standing. She chooses the ball as a treatment tool to help support the child's body weight. She applies traction to the hip joints and, over time, applies gentle force to extend and externally rotate his hips. As the child's hips extend, he is able to shift his weight from his anterior ribcage toward his lower body. This makes it easier for him to actively lift his head and look around. His visual attention assists his postural control, and this is reinforced by his mother located in front of him. The therapist begins to help the child take weight through his feet. He is in the horizontal position, but this may be a good place for the child to start. The therapist can eventually work the child into a more vertical position as the child takes over active lower extremity extension and trunk control.

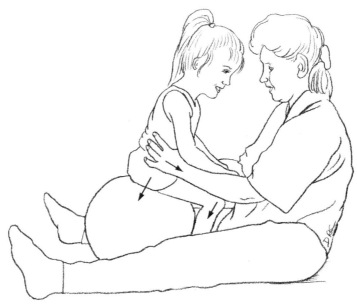

Figure 4.25   When preparing to help this child move from sit to stand, her therapist first works her feet into the best position they can achieve. This may include stretching or inhibiting activity in the shortened range of plantar flexion, followed by placing a wedge under the heels so that the hind foot contacts a weight-bearing surface to initiate anti-gravity extension. Then the therapist helps hold the lower trunk to assist its stability. This is followed by joint approximation through the lumbar facet joints to facilitate postural activity in the lower trunk. The therapist uses her forearms to provide pressure through the lower leg and heels to help the child keep contact with the weight-bearing surface as she rises.

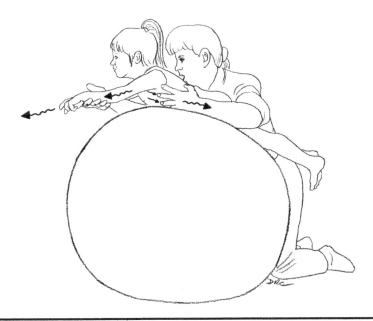

Figure 4.26   This therapist uses manual vibration to help the ribcage descend out of elevation and to help the child lengthen the arm into elbow extension. Manual vibration is performed by the therapist using small amplitude oscillations in the hand. The therapist must cocontract the arm to set up these oscillations in her hand. This is a difficult motor control task on the part of the therapist and requires practice to become proficient at it. It is well worth it because it causes the child to quickly let go of the sustained muscle holding.

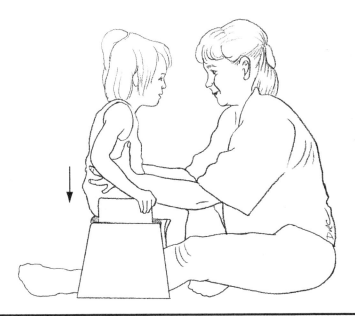

Figure 4.27   Joint approximation (compression and pressure tapping) is done through joints in their close-packed positions (the position of the joint where one articular surface is most congruent with the other—where the surfaces fit together). Joint approximation stimulates joint proprioceptors to fire, which facilitates muscle activity around the joint. Joint approximation is repeated after the therapist firmly holds the body segment to take advantage of spatial-temporal summation of sensory information.

Quadriplegia

Techniques to decrease unwanted activity in the muscles are followed immediately by techniques to increase holding and moving with muscles in the alignment needed for the functional goal.

Remember that the place this child knows how to hold with non-functional stiffness the most is in the sagittal plane (either moving between flexion and extension, or moving into just flexion or extension). Therefore, if the therapist starts work in the trunk or needs to go there after preparing the base of support, he or she often wants the trunk out of the sagittal plane. This means that the therapist works to get the trunk in rotation, usually starting with thoracic extension. This can have great results. This thoracic extension with rotation enables deeper respiration. It enables head control when upright, often when the therapist has not seen the child use head control in upright before. Thoracic extension with rotation prepares the upper extremities for moving into less scapular elevation and into more adduction with shoulder flexion and less internal rotation. It often is the key to preparing the upper body for sitting or standing. And it can be the key to beginning wider range limb movements. After accomplishing more postural control with thoracic extension with rotation, the therapist can try to go back to the sagittal plane to work if the goal for the day requires it.

Finally, in some children with hypertonic quadriplegia start with extensive work in gaining mobility, because ROM is very limited or muscle activity is sustained in a very shortened range. This is true of severely involved children as well as older children and adults. It is important to think hard about how to gain range while keeping the child active. Part of what is taught in the NDT approach is that although limited range of motion is a major problem in children with hypertonia, it is by no means their only problem. There is no time to waste in just stretching tight or overactive muscles, expecting children to somehow know how to use those muscles when there also are so many neuromuscular impairments, sensory-perceptual impairments, and impairments from other systems involved.

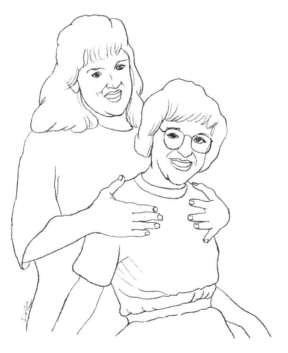

Figure 4.28 This girl is working on sustaining thoracic extension while her therapist lengthens the pectorals. The therapist opens the width of the upper chest as the hands are slowly moved along the muscle in parallel with the muscle fibers. The therapist may abduct her own fingers for additional stretch. Once she reaches the shoulders, she can move her hands laterally around the arm just below the shoulder joints as she externally rotates the shoulders. The shoulder's external rotation facilitates thoracic extension.

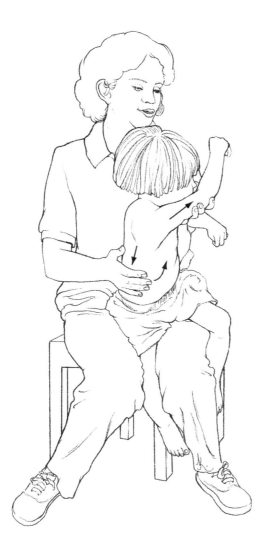

Figure 4.29   This child is working actively with visual fixation on a toy, using active assistive thoracic extension with rotation and assistance to help her terminate sustained latissimus dorsi muscle activity and/or lengthen the latissimus muscle. The therapist applies downward force at her ribcage with her right hand while assisting thoracic extension and rotation. She gives gentle sustained traction to the child's right arm with her left hand to put the latissimus muscle in its lengthened position.

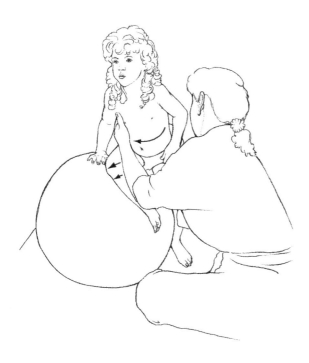

Figure 4.30   During a therapy session, this therapist assists this child into more hip extension of her left leg. She rotates her trunk to the right when it is in thoracic extension after placing her right leg against the ball in hip flexion, abduction, and external rotation. This helps the child sustain her trunk upright and shift weight over her right hip. The use of the ball provides support to the child's base of support when her hip will not abduct and externally rotate enough to reach a flat surface. The therapist then slowly extends the child's left hip. By keeping the child's trunk in rotation, excessive lumbar extension is avoided as the hip is extended. (If a tight or overactive hip flexor is stretched when the entire body is in the sagittal plane, the child responds with lumbar extension because the hip flexors attach to the lumbar spine.) The child also is now in a position to stand on her left leg as the ball supports some of her body weight.

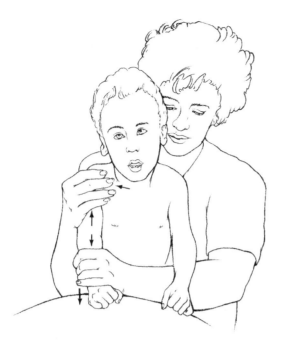

Figure 4.31 This therapist facilitates an active upper extremity support reaction. With her right hand, the therapist lengthens the pectorals to bring the shoulder into less internal rotation. As the shoulder is assisted to move back with the upper chest more open, the therapist extends the child's elbow and helps the child take weight through the arm.

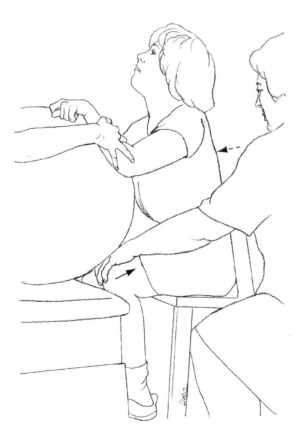

Figure 4.32 This 16-year-old girl has not stood up for many years. She has severe hamstring contractures and uses excessive lower extremity cocontraction to initiate movement among the impairments that make standing difficult for her. Her therapist uses active assistive trunk extension followed with prolonged work in as much hip flexion range as possible with her feet firmly on the floor to stretch the proximal hamstrings. She then helps the teen shift her weight forward onto her feet to practice sit to stand.

The illustrations demonstrate that it is possible and desirable to work on more than one impairment at a time. Gaining range in contracted muscles takes time—research shows that to maintain plastic elongation of connective tissue, a stretch of 20–30 minutes for a muscle group is often necessary (Miedaner & Renander, 1987). Children with cerebral palsy are known to have decreased numbers of sarcomeres in muscles that are hypoextensible (Tardieu, C., et al., 1982). Add to that the problem that experimentally immobilized muscles lose sarcomeres within days (Williams & Goldspink, 1978) and it is no wonder that therapists are concerned that clinically the same thing is likely happening in the children we treat.

Because there often are so many shortened muscles that interfere with function in a child with hypertonic quadriplegia, it would take time that therapists don't have in a treatment session to stretch these muscles (Tardieu, Lesparot, Tabary, & Bret, 1988). Then there would be no time to address the other impairments that also are interfering with function. Combining stretching with active control, more accurate perceptual information, and a better respiratory pattern involves problem solving, but it is the only way to try to address all of the impairments that interfere with function. In addition, the therapist tries to find ways for the shortened muscles to experience more range at other times of the day. Because parents and teachers often have neither the time nor the skill to stretch a muscle correctly (it can be dangerous to stretch muscles without understanding the proper technique), there have to be other options. Splinting, serial casting, night bracing, and working actively through newly gained ranges in functional skills are some of the best ways to preserve and even increase ROM.

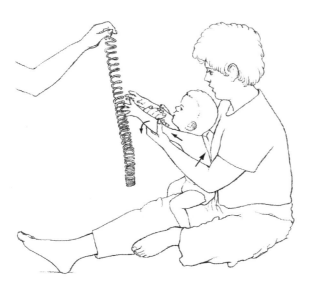

Figure 4.33 This child's mother is shown how to keep her child's latissimus and pectoral muscles working through more length as he reaches. She is shown how to support the sides of his trunk as he sits on her lap, then gently hold his shoulders in flexion with external rotation. She soon sees how much easier the reach is facilitated this way rather than by pulling on his hands, which only makes him extend his shoulders and flex his elbows as he fights back.

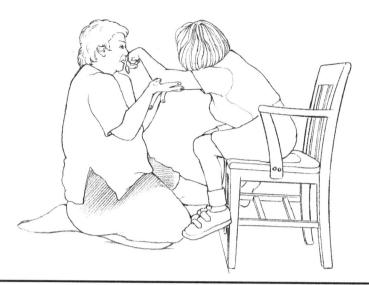

Figure 4.34 As a home program, the teenager's mother is shown how to work on ensuring that her daughter has her weight on her feet before rising to stand (Figure 4.32). She works with her daughter on exaggerating the degree of hip flexion to assure that her center of mass comes forward over her feet. She works with her daughter on this part of the sit to stand transfer at first without trying to help her stand up. As they practice, the teenager assists leaning forward and learns to move around her hip joints rather than trying to round her thoracic spine to lean forward.

After beginning with one of these three approaches—widening the base of support, working on head and trunk alignment and postural activity, or working to gain range of motion—think about how to get this child to move. This usually works best when keeping the child's trunk out of the sagittal plane, at least to begin with, while facilitating wider movements of the limbs.

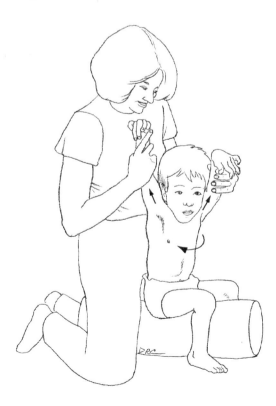

Figure 4.35 This child is visually engaged with his mother's face as she sits in front of him and sings (mother not pictured). His therapist brings his arms overhead to inhibit shoulder internal rotation and thoracic flexion while facilitating active assistive thoracic extension with rotation. The bolster the child sits on keeps his left leg in place. Because his trunk is rotated to the right over the left thigh, his left hip joint is abducted and externally rotated.

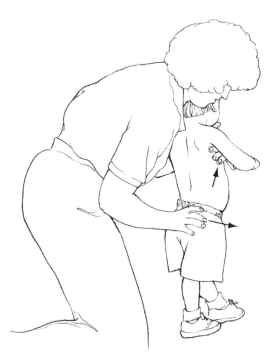

Figure 4.36 In standing, it often is easier to facilitate a step from the stride position rather than starting with the feet side by side. Part of this may be that by placing the trunk in thoracic extension with rotation as a starting position, the child cannot use the familiar straight sagittal plane flexion and extension movements that he is familiar with to initiate movement and the therapist can help him try a new strategy. Another reason may be that active trunk rotation facilitates active extremity dissociation (interlimb coordination).

The work helps the child learn to move with less voluntary stiffness of the limbs while keeping the trunk active posturally. This prepares for learning new skills for function. This is where the therapist can emphasize movement transitions in treatment because they are so hard for children with hypertonia to make. These are often the functional goals therapists have set for the child, so that the therapist may need eventually to start working back toward the sagittal plane and/or to decrease the wider range movements. This can be a difficult place in the treatment progression, as it is easy for the child to stiffen and return to familiar stiff postures.

These movement transitions can include the ones we easily think of, such as rolling, getting in and out of sitting, and standing up. But there also are many times when small, subtle shifts in the center of mass and base of support are necessary to perform a skill that can be described as movement transition. Therapists also must think about working for the larger transitional movements in smaller pieces, such as working to shift the weight in sitting just enough to facilitate a support reaction of an arm prior to turning to get down to the floor from a chair.

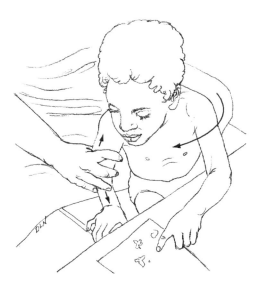

Figure 4.37 This child works to push a puzzle piece into a puzzle board. His occupational therapist guides him into thoracic rotation toward the right. With thoracic extension and rotation, upper extremity weight bearing on the right arm is easily facilitated. His therapist supports his right elbow to assist its graded flexion/extension control as he takes more, then less weight through the right arm as he reaches with his left and moves his trunk.

Quadriplegia

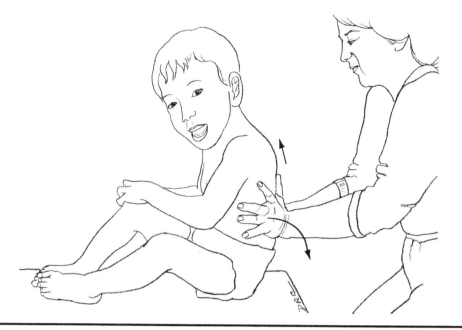

Figure 4.38   This child's mother is learning how to help her child lift his foot to put a shoe on. She learns that he must first shift his weight toward the back of his base of support in order to unweight his feet. His therapist teaches her to make sure that she helps him keep his thoracic spine actively extended while he shifts back. His mother uses her hands to assist thoracic extension while helping him tilt back and hold with his abdominal muscles.

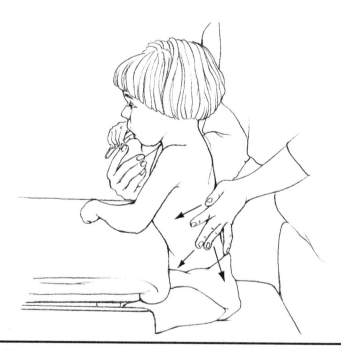

Figure 4.39   Many children with hypertonia have difficulty bringing an eating utensil to their mouths. To reach forward, they often flex in the thoracic spine, which does not efficiently move their centers of mass forward. Here, this child's therapist shows and assists her to both hold thoracic extension and move forward around her hip joints as she brings the spoon to her mouth.

As the child and therapist work, care should be taken to ensure the best possible alignment of all body segments for the most efficient use of the ability to initiate, sustain, and terminate desirable muscle activity. Also, if the child can keep the trunk active and moving as needed for a skill without increasing the stiffness of the limbs, breath holding as a way to gain stability decreases, and is replaced by trunk postural control.

C A S E   S T U D Y

Look at a case study to follow an assessment and treatment plan for a child with hypertonic quadriplegia. The child is a 7-year-old girl who is seeing her speech pathologist with her parents in attendance at an outpatient clinic. The parents estimate that the child uses more than 100 words but she cannot speak more than two words per breath. She initiates voicing with eye, cervical, lumbar, and lower extremity extension. Her vocal quality is strained and hoarse. She quickly runs out of air and has to terminate all her extension (she looks very stiff as she talks, then slumps in her chair for a minute), then starts the process of extension through her body again with the next breath to say one or two more words.

In the clinical assessment, her parents feel that their daughter is comfortable and is performing typically in her communication skills. Her speech pathologist may find that in addition to the above observations, the child speaks an average of two words per breath and speaks no more than 30 words per minute. This does not enable her to enter conversations with many people, adults or children. It is likely that many people would not be patient enough to wait until she says all that she wants to say. In addition, the child has many articulation errors that make her speech difficult to understand.

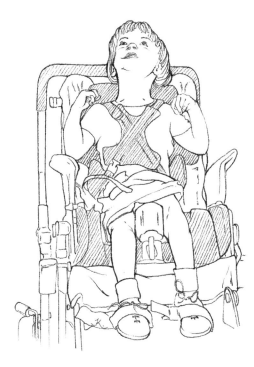

Figure 4.40 This child with spastic athetosis initiates voicing by pushing out her exhalation with lumbar, cervical, and eye extension. As she does this, her limbs stiffen with cocontraction.

The parents and therapist decide that one important goal is that the child speak faster and be able to say more words per breath. One treatment goal, then, is that the child is able to say four words per breath at least five times during the session. The therapist may decide to further evaluate the child's ribcage structure and muscular activity of the trunk for breath support. On observation, the child shows several impairments. Her ribcage is elevated, with the ribs more horizontally positioned than should be present in 7-year-olds. She has limited passive mobility into thoracic extension and can be rotated passively only about 20° to each side. She is a belly breather with little to no ribcage movement both with and without voicing. In addition, her postural muscles, including thoracic extensors and abdominal muscles, are inactive in control of her trunk. Her hips are positioned and actively held in slight flexion, adduction, and internal rotation in her seating system or when held on someone's lap.

The therapist may decide that the child's ribcage needs to descend passively out of elevation, and that the child needs to increase passive mobility into thoracic extension and rotation and become more active posturally in her trunk. If the therapist can help the child hold the trunk and ribcage actively with thoracic extension, abdominal muscles, and intercostals as the position of the ribcage changes, then the effects of treatment have the possibility of carryover as she practices talking, especially if the treatment session is followed by a good home program.

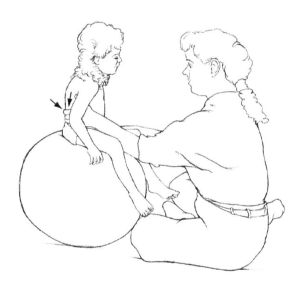

Figure 4.41   This child actively will hold trunk and cervical extension above her therapist's hands as her therapist brings her ribcage out of elevation and helps her into more thoracic extension as the arrows indicate.

As the therapist, you may decide that the child must learn a new movement synergy for initiating voicing. Begin by asking her to look at her tummy as you facilitate a chin tuck by tilting her upper body toward the back of her base of support. Help her keep the ribcage down out of elevation, rotate her slightly to keep the intercostals out of a shortened range, and use manual vibration as she exhales and voices to help prolong and grade the exhalation. Practice this for the remainder of the treatment session.

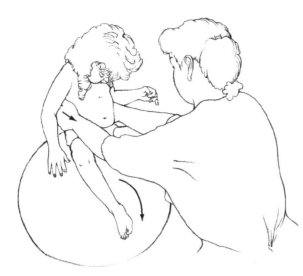

Figure 4.42 The therapist helps this child become active in sustaining both the trunk postural extensors and flexors. She assists thoracic extension with hands on the child's lower ribcage posteriorly and shifting her center of mass forward. Then she helps hold the trunk in extension as she tips the child back toward the back of her base of support. It is important to tip the child back by keeping the trunk extended and hips flexed (like tilting a chair on its back legs). The therapist moves the ball the child sits on toward herself as she tilts the child back. This keeps the child close to her for safety.

As a home program, ask her parents to seat their child on their lap. Show them how to open (abduct) her hips and turn them out, then how to support her trunk erect. Ask them to hold her shoulders so that they do not ele-vate and pull forward (inhibition of shoulder complex elevation and shoulder joint internal rotation). In this position, they can read a story together and talk about the pictures in the story.

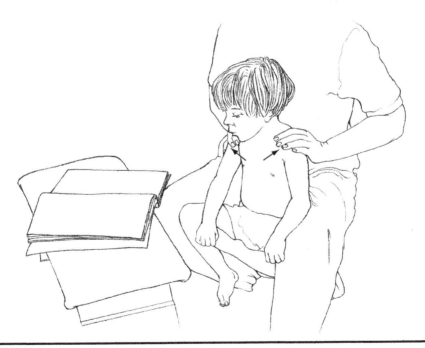

Figure 4.43 As the child and her parents practice actively holding the child's trunk in more extension, her parents help position her shoulder complex out of its elevated position and bring the shoulder joints into a position of more flexion and external rotation. This position also lengthens the pectoral muscles.

Quadriplegia

Diplegia

Typical Posture and Movement Strategies

Head, neck, tongue, and eyes

The child with diplegia may have variable development of control of the head, neck, tongue, and eyes. Those who have more involvement in the upper body may develop head, cervical spine, tongue, and jaw control similar to a child with quadriplegia. (The difference between a child with diplegia and a child with quadriplegia depends on who is making the diagnosis. Therefore, a child with upper body involvement may be diagnosed as diplegic because the lower body involvement is so much more severe. The same child could be diagnosed as quadriplegic by someone else because the entire body is involved, even if the lower body is more involved than the upper.)

In children whose lesions result in less upper body involvement, it is not uncommon to see fairly typical early development of control and coordination in this area of the body. They are able to initiate, sustain, and terminate muscle activity well; to coordinate a variety of movement synergies that are functional; to time movements well; and to use sensory-perceptual information effectively (except for vision). Many have trouble coordinating vision with movement or making the eyes work together. Children with diplegia often have early problems with strabismus and other primary impairments that interfere with smooth visual pursuits and eyes that work together. This may or may not affect early development of head control, but if no obvious difficulties are noted at this time, it is wise to continue to monitor this closely. Visual problems may be overlooked when the problems of lower body control are so much more obvious. However, if visual problems are never addressed, the older child and

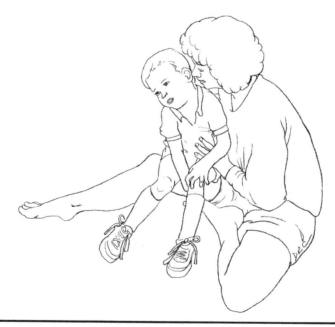

Figure 4.44 This child holds his head tilted to the right. Although at first glance it appears that he does not have good head control, careful observation shows that he holds his head erect until he tries to visually focus on books or toys brought closer than 24" in front of his face.

adult may find that this eventually prevents them from achieving important functions. For example, a teenager may have great difficulty learning to drive, not necessarily because of lower body control, but because of poor vision. Other children, whose teachers feel they could keep up academically with grade-level work, fall behind because reading becomes so slow. Some may find it hard to look at the chalkboard or computer screen and then at a paper at a different focal length while completing an assignment. Another child may hold her head in such an awkward, tiring position to stabilize her eyes to work smoothly that she is too slow in completing her work.

Other problems with head and trunk control may develop later when the child needs to use his lower body as the base of support and as a place of stability from which to initiate movement. Therefore, it is not unusual to see an infant or very young child with diplegia show fairly good head posture and control in all positions he can assume or use. But when the lower body needs to control the base of support and initiate movement and is unable to, the child often learns to use his head to try to initiate weight shifting or to hold his head in abnormal alignment because the lower body is so abnormally aligned. To the parent, the child is now getting worse or is showing new problems. Of course, there is concern.

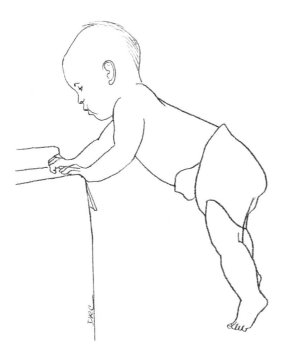

Figure 4.45 This baby was thought to be developing normally until she began supported standing and pull to standing. She could only stand with her hips and ankles plantar flexed, then began internally rotating her hips soon after she began standing. Until then, her upper body postures and movements appeared normal. Now, if she were to try to shift her weight in standing to begin supported stepping, she would likely move her cervical spine into end range extension in an attempt to shift her center of mass over her feet. When she does that, her head movements look *abnormal*. The more she has to compensate with her upper body for what her lower body will not do, the more *abnormal* her upper body appears.

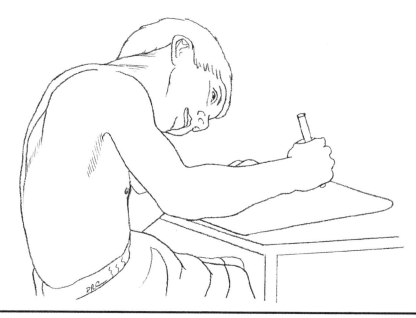

Figure 4.46 This 10-year-old uses his thoracic flexion and a forward positioned head to attempt to bring himself forward in his chair to see his writing assignment. His hips are adducted and internally rotated, and he sustains holding in this position with the effort of writing. In standing, he holds his head erect and his upper thoracic spine extended.

Functionally, the child with diplegia often has good head contol until head alignment is affected by the lower body and the child tries to use the head as a substitute for lower body movement. Head control can be affected early on, or not until later. Head position can be altered by poor control of vision and appear as poor head control.

Imagine some of the disabilities. A 10-month-old shows adequate control of this area of the body when he is in supine, prone, or sitting on his mother's lap. When he sits on the floor, however, he cannot look at toys on the floor or guide his reach with vision because his cervical spine is extended to try to keep him upright in sitting when his back is so rounded. A 2-year-old can hold her head up and rotate as needed for the skills she can do—creep on all fours, pull to stand, feed herself with a fork, and talk. But when she wants to put simple puzzles together, color with crayons, or look at a book that her mother reads to her, she tilts her head to the left and then cannot always complete the activity visually or with her hands. A 16-year-old can walk independently, dress himself slowly, function independently at school, and work in the summers at a concession stand, but cannot pass a driver's test because of his vision.

Thoracic spine, ribcage, and upper extremities

For children with diplegia, this area of the body develops in a variety of ways. Some show the ability to use upper-extremity weight bearing in ways that are similar to children developing normally. The difference is that children with diplegia seem to retain more shoulder complex elevation, perhaps as a way to use the more superficial muscles for control because the lower trunk musculature is not working as efficiently as it does in children developing without CP. When this shoulder complex elevation is retained and prolonged, the results are that the child learns to push the arms down against a surface (the upper body can initiate, sustain, and terminate effectively, grade cocontraction, and use a variety of functional synergies), but shoulder extension and internal rotation are seen more frequently because of the shoulder complex elevation. The elbow tends to stay more flexed with the forearm pronated with this proximal posturing. The thoracic spine extends with this weight bearing, but in the upper thoracic area only. Many children with diplegia show strong upper thoracic extension, but a mildly rounded lower thoracic area. To extend the lower thoracic area in development, the child seems to need to grade upper extremity and trunk movements against a surface, lifting the chest up higher as the elbows extend with shoulder flexion. Shifting the weight with trunk rotation incorporated into the movement also helps. Shoulder complex elevation, even mildly, affects the alignment of the serratus anterior and rhomboids, making them less efficient as scapular stabilizers. The rounding of the lower thoracic area prevents full development of trunk rotation and later development of overhead reach.

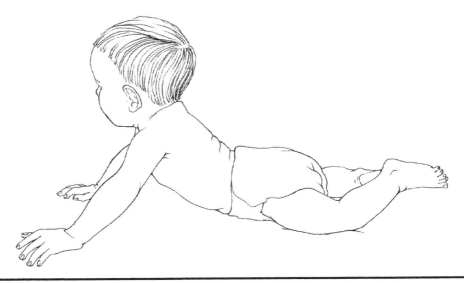

Figure 4.47 This 6-month-old with no developmental impairments is able to begin grading elbow flexion and extension as she pushes against the floor in prone. Her shoulders are in flexion and she actively extends her entire thoracic spine.

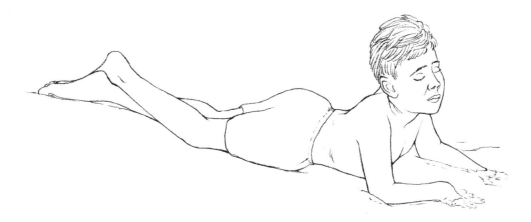

Figure 4.48 This 8-year-old with diplegia enjoys a day at the beach. As he lies in the water, he props on his forearms. His shoulder complex is slightly elevated with shoulder internal rotation. His upper thoracic spine is extended and the lower thoracic spine is in a position of extension. But because he cannot bring his shoulders into flexion with neutral external rotation and push up with elbow extension and with active abdominal holding, his lower thoracic spine does not actively extend.

Diplegia

Lower thoracic extension is needed for stability in overhead reach, erect sitting, and alignment for the efficient use of lower trunk weight shifting. These often are skills with which children with diplegia have great difficulty.

Some children with diplegia have more trunk involvement, and they tend to retain more thoracic flexion throughout the spine. They also have poor upper-extremity weight-bearing skills with the shoulder complex very elevated, the shoulders extended and internally rotated, the elbows flexed, forearms pronated, and hands flexed, with very little variability to this posture. These children have much more ribcage elevation, lower rib flaring, and rigidity to the ribcage than the children already described. Because their lower bodies are much more involved than their upper bodies, they often are considered diplegic, although their trunks are much more like children who have quadriplegia.

For all children with diplegia, no matter how this area of the body initially presents, posture and function can, and often do, worsen, as the lower body becomes responsible for base of support and for initiation of movement. This is just as it was described in the section on head, neck, tongue, and eyes on page 104. For example, a child may be able to use his arms for support, to reach and manipulate some toys, and to finger feed. But then he spends more time in sitting and standing with very inefficient alignment of the lower body. This alignment directly impacts the alignment of the upper body. The child also uses the upper body to substitute for what the lower body will not do. He may do this by holding longer with upper body postures and by stiffening his arms. The result is that the upper body looks more *spastic* as it voluntarily works overtime to compensate for the lower body.

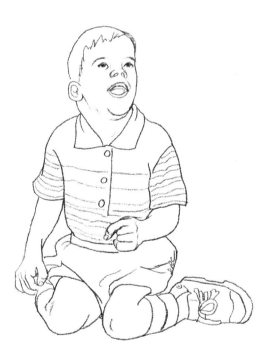

Figure 4.49 W-sitting is an option that many children with diplegia use. It enables them to use their hip flexion, adduction, and internal rotation positioning, but provides a wider base of support than when using the same hip position with the legs and feet in front of the child. On careful observation, the therapist notes that this sitting posture includes thoracic and lumbar flexion with excessive cervical extension. The inability to move the lower trunk and lower extremities in this position limits range of reach with the arms and even limits smooth visual pursuits as the child uses cervical extension only.

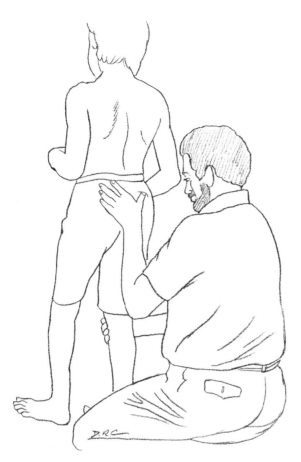

Figure 4.50 In standing, the child uses shoulder extension to assist trunk extension. He has a great deal of difficulty activating lower lumbar and hip extension (his therapist is helping him do this now). Holding the arms in shoulder extension as a way to assist lower body extension severely limits use of the arms; in standing this child cannot reach, carry, or hold anything. His arms have become part of his postural system functionally, which eliminates the reaching, grasping, exploring, and manipulation skills for which the human arms are designed.

Functionally, the problems that result are from incomplete extension and rotation of the thoracic spine; incomplete shoulder flexion and external rotation; incomplete ability to horizontally adduct the arms; and incomplete elbow extension, forearm supination, and wrist and finger extension. Problems also seem to appear and progress when the upper trunk and extremities work to compensate for what the lower body cannot do. Therefore, arms may get stiffer with effort as the lower body cannot shift weight. The thoracic spine may increase its flexion as the pectorals and rectus abdominus work hard to pull the center of mass forward when the hips are unable to do so in sitting and standing.

Disabilities that result from these functional limitations include some of the following:

- A 9-month-old is unable to hold a toy with both hands at midline as he sits on his mother's lap because he has to use his arms to assist trunk control. He also cannot hold many toys because his forearms remain in some degree of pronation with wrist flexion, ulnar deviation, finger and thumb flexion, and thumb adduction.

- A 4-year-old is able to use bunny hopping to move about the floor (upper extremities moving in phase with each other, and lower extremities also moving in phase with each other, a pattern requiring basic flexion and extension synergies only). She can get in and out of small chairs and benches pulling with her upper body as she drags her legs behind her. She can feed herself using fingers and a fork, but has trouble with a spoon. She can stack blocks, put together simple puzzles, use crayons with a static tripod grasp, but cannot dress her dolls, draw a square or triangle, or begin to cut with scissors.

Diplegia

- A 12-year-old can walk with crutches, use a computer, dress and undress herself except for back fasteners and shoe tying, and use writing for her schoolwork when time is not a factor, but cannot fix her own hair or use writing for most classroom assignments because she is so slow.

Lower trunk

Although children with diplegia may vary in the use of the upper trunk and upper extremities, the lower trunk is remarkably similar in most such children. Typically, they use the superficial lumbar extensors with the hip flexors as the primary, if not only, synergy to control the ribcage on the pelvis. There is little or no use of the abdominal muscles as a group to stabilize the ribcage to the pelvis, provide support for respiration, or limit the movement of the center of mass. There is little use of the hip extensors, primarily the gluteus maximus, to control the hips in any position. There seems to be little variability in the way the lower trunk is controlled—only the severity of the lack of the synergistic use of the abdominal muscles and hip extensors seems to vary.

Especially in prone and standing, the upper lumbar spine is positioned in end-range extension while the hips are flexed to various degrees. This upper lumbar extension can be so severe that the child seems to develop abnormal mobility at several levels, usually from the lower thoracic spine to the upper lumbar spine. This is a place in the spine where mobility is easily gained (watch gymnasts and dancers). One reason is biomechanical—the facet joints change planes abruptly at about T-12 from the coronal to the sagittal plane, thereby offering this area mobility in rotation as well as flexion/extension. Another reason is that the attachments of the diaphragm and iliopsoas influence the upper lumbar spine, which is pulled into extension as these muscles shorten and/or sustain the midrange contractions typical of children with diplegia.

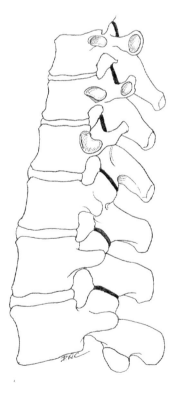

Figure 4.51 Note the change in plane orientation of the facet joints at T-12. The facet joints of the thoracic spine lie primarily in the coronal plane, enabling rotation as the main movement. The facet joints in the lumbar spine lie primarily in the sagittal plane, enabling primarily flexion/extension movement.

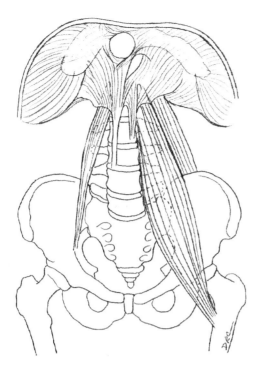

Figure 4.52 The central tendon of the diaphragm inserts into the lumbar vertebral bodies while the psoas major originates laterally on the vertebral bodies. (The psoas also blends into a portion of the diaphragm.) These muscles are often tight and overactive in children with diplegia, contributing another factor in the excessive lumbar extension.

As the child is pulled into strong upper lumbar extension with some degree of hip flexion, the abdominal muscles are overlengthened, further weakening the use of this group. The end-range extension also prevents rotation from occurring higher in the thoracic spine—when the spine is in end range flexion or extension it is difficult if not impossible biomechanically to rotate the spine. Therefore, the child has to move the trunk in patterns of flexion/extension, further inhibiting use of abdominal obliques and intercostals for control of the ribcage and lower trunk.

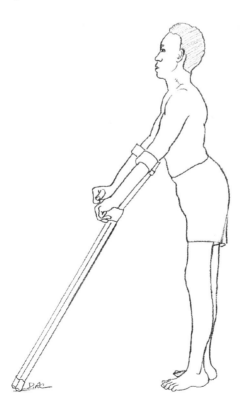

Figure 4.53 This 14-year-old stands with the trunk and lower extremity postures described on page 110. His trunk extension is most prominent in the cervical and thoracolumbar areas with his hips in flexion, adduction, and internal rotation.

Some children also use lateral flexion with the majority of the mobility occurring at the lower thoracic/upper lumbar area only, rather than throughout the thoracic spine. This may develop because the child cannot use the lower trunk to initiate weight shifting, just as in the child described previously. From a position of upper lumbar extension, the child learns to lean the trunk in the coronal plane, pivoting around the upper lumbar area. This may occur as a compensation in children with poor hip joint development and, therefore, poor biomechanics for hip abductor use. There is the strong possibility that the vertebrae in this area of the spine become abnormally shaped and enable mobility, especially laterally, that is not possible in the normally shaped spine.

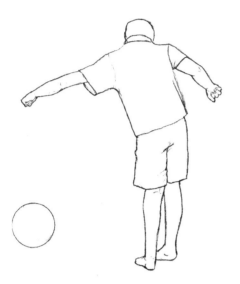

Figure 4.54 This 5-year-old child with diplegia is going to kick the ball with his right foot. To shift weight onto his left lower extremity in preparation for the kick, he laterally flexes his trunk to the left (shifts upper trunk over lower trunk). This indicates a probable lack of the ability to stabilize the hip joint with the hip abductors.

Most children with diplegia develop either the flexion/extension strategy of shifting weight, using strong extension in the upper lumbar area in prone and standing, or the lateral flexion strategy, still with the upper lumbar spine in a position of extension. Sometimes the child uses the same strategy to move in sitting and sometimes she succumbs to gravity and sinks into flexion. In either instance, the upper and lower trunk do not *connect*—they do not work together to control the center of mass for balancing, control of respiration, or control of weight shifting. This becomes a problem for all therapists working with children with diplegia, not just physical therapists.

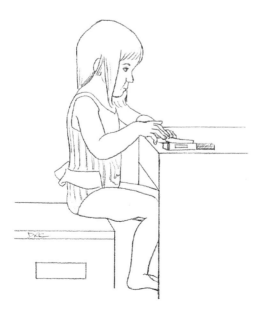

Figure 4.55 This 3-year-old who is developing without neuromuscular impairments moves her entire trunk by flexing at her hips while the trunk is extended to reach or look forward.

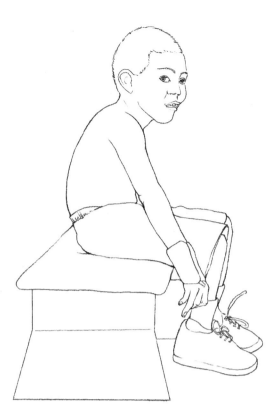

Figure 4.56 This 4-year-old collapses into trunk flexion in sitting. As he tries to reach forward, he cannot move his center of mass forward to a more stable position within his base of support by using trunk extension. He therefore tries to use cervical extension to do so, but it is ineffective. One major influence in his inability to reach forward is his inability to sit erect—he cannot lift his arm here because if he tried he would fall over backward.

Functionally, the child with diplegia has a great deal of difficulty with any of the multitude of skills that require controlled mobility of the lower trunk. The child has trouble controlling this area of the body, which is responsible for upright balance, mobility through space, and coordinating respiration with phonation.

The disabilities of a 12-month-old with diplegia may include that she cannot move about on the floor as her upper lumbar spine sustains end-range extension while her lower extremities stiffen as she lifts her upper body in prone. Therefore, she cannot shift her weight to separate her legs (actively separating the extremities from each other requires control of trunk rotation) to crawl or creep. When placed in sitting, however, she sinks into trunk flexion with insufficient hip flexion and cannot say the several words that she is capable of when held in her mother's lap.

A 5-year-old walks with a walker, but only at home or in the classroom because the excessive movement of his center of mass in gait causes him to expend about 70% more energy than a child who walks normally. He also cannot climb stairs independently, even with a rail.

A 17-year-old who walks independently and negotiates stairs and curbs still cannot keep up with his friends when they go to the mall or ball games. He worries that he will be limited in choosing a college based on distance he has to walk.

The pelvic girdle and lower extremities

Because of the lesions that cause diplegia, there is a marked discrepancy between control of the upper body and that of the lower body. The lower extremities show limited synergies for use in function; a poor ability to grade cocontraction and reciprocal inhibition with excessive cocontraction often used; a poor ability to terminate sustained muscle activity; and abnormal timing of muscle contractions. These impairments are seen to a much lesser degree in the upper body. In addition, secondary impairments in the musculoskeletal system can develop rapidly. This is because the child with diplegia, as opposed to the child with quadriplegia, finds some way to get into sitting and standing relatively soon. The alignment and control of sitting and standing can be very abnormal, so that gravity and external forces quickly deform bones, help shorten muscles, and malalign joints. The hips are almost always pulled into flexion, adduction, and internal rotation with little effective opposition from their antagonists (see the section on quadriplegia for more details). This sets the child up for hip dysplasia and early subluxation or dislocation. It also narrows the base of support in all positions, which makes learning upright trunk control more difficult.

The medial hamstrings are the muscles that seem most responsible for the hip internal rotation. They also are knee flexors. Therefore, it is not uncommon to see children in some degree of knee flexion in all their postures. Some children with diplegia show very stiffly extended knees. In these children, there usually is less of an internal rotation component to their hips and more of a flexion component. It is with this posture that the rectus femoris can exert strong influence as a hip flexor and knee extensor.

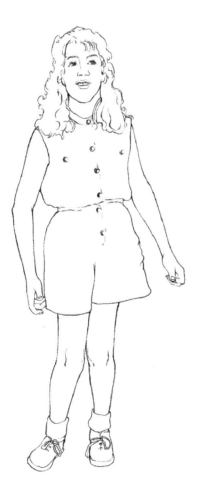

Figure 4.57 This 12-year-old learned to walk fairly erect, working hard to overcome and lessen many impairments. She stands asymmetrically here, with most weight on her left foot. Her hips are slightly flexed, and the right hip shows both adduction and internal rotation posturing. Her knee also is slightly flexed.

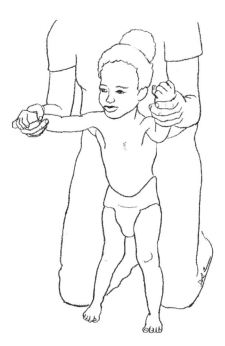

Figure 4.58 This child with ataxia shows one of the same patterns in the lower extremities that some children with diplegia use. Her hips are very flexed with her center of mass toward the back or even behind her base of support. She strongly sustains contraction of her quadriceps femoris and possibly her hamstrings. A child with diplegia may do all of this with more hip adduction and internal rotation as well.

In both cases, the ankles assume a plantar-flexed position because of a combination of many factors. The plantar flexors are a group of muscles that have a large cross sectional area compared with their antagonists. The gastrocnemious muscle also is a two-joint muscle, and its primary antagonist, the anterior tibialis, is not. In addition, children with diplegia almost always find a way to stand up with help, and so ground reaction forces, as well as a need to balance, bias the use of the plantar flexors (this last consideration does not happen in the upper extremity).

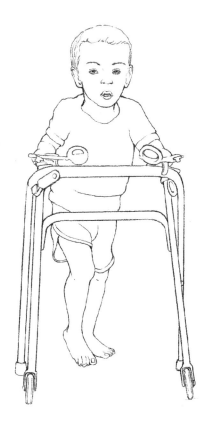

Figure 4.59 As this child stands at his walker, several factors influence the bias toward ankle plantar flexion. First, he uses sustained lower extremity cocontraction, and the plantar flexors are much larger in cross sectional area than the dorsiflexors, so the ankle assumes a plantar flexed position. Secondly, as he leans forward on his walker and cannot stand erect using a controlled trunk with postural hip extension, he pitches forward on his toes as a way to move the center of mass forward. Finally, as he steps from this alignment, the ground reaction force stretches a shortened range, overactive gastrocnemius, allowing the muscle only concentric contractions with little joint movement.

Functionally, the child is limited to the use of hip flexion, adduction, internal rotation, a varying position of the knee, and ankle plantar flexion with a variable foot position. Other synergies to control base of support and movement either do not develop or develop to a very limited degree. This is why so many children with diplegia choose W-sitting as the only way they can floor sit. W-sitting enables the hips, knees, and ankles to assume these limited positions while providing a wide base of support. It often is the only way the child can sit and have a stable enough base of support to free the hands for play.

Remember that these synergies are limited not only as primary impairments, but because a number of neuromuscular, musculoskeletal, and to a lesser degree, perceptual impairments influence each other to limit function. For example, primary neuromuscular impairments influence the hip to assume strong flexion, adduction, and internal rotation. This places the hip abductor in poor alignment for effective contraction to stabilize the hip laterally. Flexion, adduction, and internal rotation working unopposed also deform the hip in a way that further compromises hip abductor function (Arnold, Komattu, & Delp, 1997; Cornell, 1995). Then the child has to compensate, usually with an upper body weight shift, to substitute for the ineffective hip abductors. Over time, the perception of how to shift weight becomes familiar with practice, so that if the child is given a more stable hip surgically or in therapy, he doesn't automatically know a different way to shift his weight, even if it is more energy efficient.

Let's predict some of the common disabilities. A 2-year-old can pull to stand at furniture, but cannot walk around it or walk independently. He also can only W-sit on the floor. At circle time in preschool, all his classmates sit tailor style. A 5-year-old can walk independently, but cannot negotiate stairs or curbs. He likes to go out to the playground at recess, but cannot get on and off most of the equipment. A 10-year-old with more severe involvement can walk in the classroom and at home with a walker, but cannot get up and down to the walker without assistance. She also cannot manage any lower extremity dressing independently and needs help with clothing in the bathroom. She speaks in short phrases only, with her lumbar spine extending as her legs stiffen when she pushes out the air with every word. Therefore, she is unable to enter conversations except for dialogue with one familiar person at a time.

General Treatment Strategies

No matter what your therapy specialty is—physical, occupational, or speech—you probably will find that you must start your treatment in the same place to accomplish your functional goal. There are two areas to be targeted in treatment of children with diplegia in preparation for more diverse practice of skills. One is working to gain stability of the lower trunk with more synergy options. Therefore, work to gain activity in the abdominal muscles—all of them—with the entire trunk in a position of extension. This is how the abdominal muscles work functionally for most skills—the trunk must be active or supported in extension to stabilize the spine before the abdominal muscles can actively stabilize the lower trunk anteriorly (Bly, 1994).

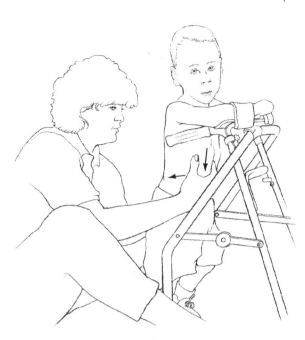

Figure 4.60a As this child learns to use his walker, his therapist supports his abdominal muscles. She helps align his lower trunk so that he uses extension of his trunk, but not end range thoracolumbar extension only. She helps the base of the ribcage descend and angles force diagonally toward the hips to help the child maintain trunk extension with hip extension. Her support on his abdominal muscles also assists him in stability of his lower trunk so that he can better control *connection* between the upper and lower body.

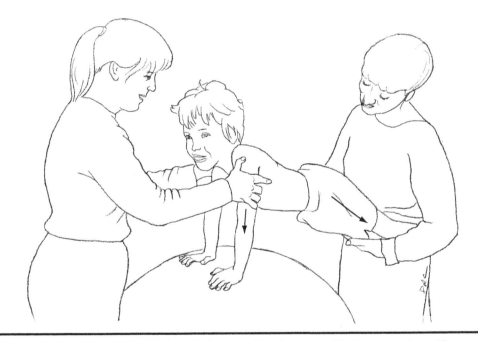

Figure 4.60b This child with diplegia has better trunk control and options for movement than the child in Figure 4.60a. However, he still does not always hold his lower trunk with adequate postural control for skills such as breathing efficiently while running, for stair climbing, and for dressing himself while standing. His therapists support him in shoulder complex stability on his ribcage and in hip extension with external rotation. As he actively supports himself in this position, his abdominal muscles become part of the postural synergy he uses. Frequently, sustaining shoulder flexion with external rotation and horizontal adduction, especially with weight bearing or a distal external load, facilitates postural holding with the abdominal muscles.

Then work with the child to hold postures that require trunk and hip extensor activity with abdominal activity. The activity that you want is for the lower trunk to stay still while the limbs move. This can be extremely difficult, but absolutely necessary to develop many functions.

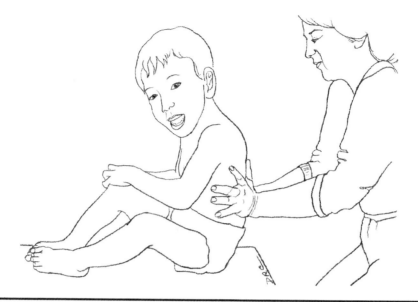

Figure 4.61   This child's mother is learning how to help her child lift his foot to put a shoe on. She learns that he must first shift his weight toward the back of his base of support to unweight his feet. His therapist teaches her to make sure that she helps him keep his thoracic spine actively extended while he shifts back. His mother uses her hands to assist thoracic extension while helping him tilt back and hold with his abdominal muscles.

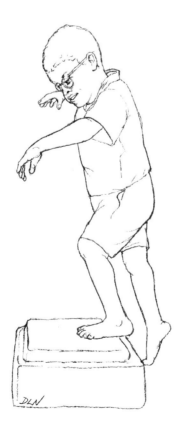

Figure 4.62   This child is using trunk and lower extremity extensor muscle groups to rise onto the step. However, to initially lift and place his foot on the step, he has to shift weight back to the opposite heel. This is likely to require the extension in the trunk and weight bearing leg, but also abdominal stability and hip flexion control in the foot that is being placed on the step. The need for abdominal and hip flexor control increases with the height of the step.

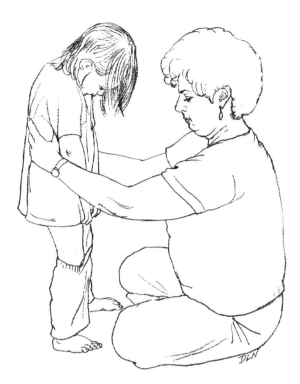

Figure 4.63 This child is learning to pull up her pants in standing. Her therapist supports her thoracic spine in extension and gives repetitive joint approximation through her lower body for somatosensory information. As the child looks and reaches down, the abdominal muscles may be a part of the trunk flexion used to reach as well as be part of postural trunk support.

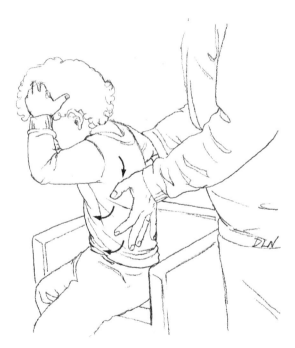

Figure 4.64 In therapy, this child is working for functional skills that involve care of her hair. The therapist first helps her extend and rotate her trunk to assist overhead reach. Later in the therapy session, they will return to a symmetrical sitting posture and work to lift the arms overhead where the child will likely have more difficulty activating lower trunk extension to get the arms overhead. In addition, once the arms are overhead, the center of mass may shift toward the back of the base of support, which could require abdominal activity to prevent falling backward.

The lower trunk is a place where the center of mass is located, so it should not be moving excessively. Consider also how often the entire trunk needs to move as a well-coordinated whole in function. This is something that children with diplegia have an extremely hard time doing. One of the biggest problems they have in movement is that the upper and lower trunk do not work together—it is as if they are two separate halves with no connection in direction of movement and coordination. So you must work to gain that connection of the upper and lower trunk for many different functions.

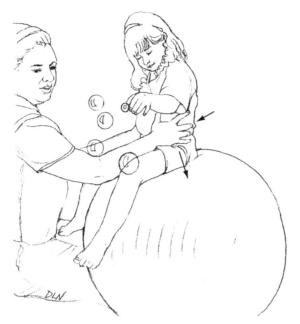

Figure 4.65 As this child reaches forward, her therapist assists lumbar extension and active hip flexion rather than the midthoracic flexion with lack of hip stability against the support surface the child typically attempts.

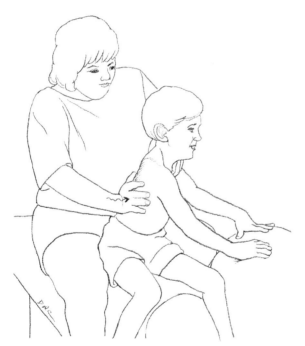

Figure 4.66 This child's speech pathologist uses manual vibration as the child speaks to help decrease breath holding and increase the length of exhalation. She also assists trunk rotation as he speaks to help grade the exhalation. She wants him to increase the number of syllables he can say per breath for the goal of answering questions promptly and quickly in class.

Although this section on treatment began by discussing the controlled stability of the lower trunk and its movement in harmony with the upper trunk, it is impossible to achieve this if the base of support is so abnormal that trunk activity is inhibited by malalignment or overactivity of lower extremity muscles, or both. Therefore, you must continue looking back and forth between the base of support and lower trunk activity. In some children it is impossible to begin work on the lower trunk until they have established a better base of support. In others, the way to establish a better base of support, that is, to get them to let go of excessive sustained activity of some of the lower extremity muscles, is to work on establishing a more stable lower trunk. Try both ways until you find the place that that child needs to start establishing change for more function.

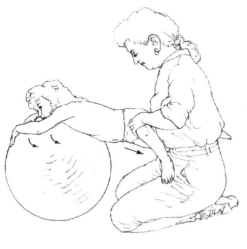

Figure 4.67a This therapist works to increase the range of hip external rotation in this child. She incorporates trunk extension and rotation into the alignment, which makes lower extremity dissociation easier. The child actively holds the ball to assist activity in the trunk.

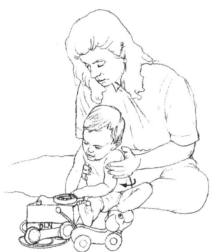

Figure 4.67b One way to increase range at the hip is to move the trunk over a fixed hip. By assisting active trunk rotation with reaching to the right, the therapist can increase mobility in the left hip if it remains or is helped to remain in a fixed position. An important part of this child's treatment is the support to the left thigh by the therapist's leg. Since his abduction range is limited, providing a support surface for the range he has allows him to terminate holding of his leg in the air, and rely on external support for stability. Now his thigh is part of his base of support.

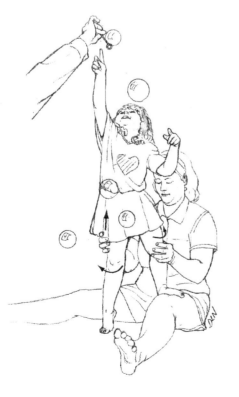

Figure 4.67c This child is working to learn to jump from the floor. When she attempts to jump now, she internally rotates her hips and does not yet have enough strength in her plantar flexors. Her therapist assists active plantar flexion by externally rotating her hip and helping her lift part of her body weight. She also externally rotates the other hip to help the child use her gluteals to extend the hips.

Once the child's base of support is more stable and well-aligned, and the lower trunk is increasingly active and can better hold the center of mass stable, you can work more toward the functional skill. For example, a speech pathologist may need the child to be able to say more words per exhalation or need alignment of the oral structures for feeding. In a child with diplegia, it may be necessary to establish a better base of support with the lower extremities less stiff, and a more active lower trunk with abdominal muscles assisting breath support for each skill. For an occupational therapist, the goal of combing hair or putting on socks while seated may require the same work in the lower body before more specific work related to the skill. For a physical therapist, the goals of moving in and out of sitting, standing and walking with an assistive device, and climbing stairs again have the prerequisites of a well-aligned, controlled base of support and a posturally active lower trunk.

Always remember that many children with diplegia have complex visual impairments that can severely limit their function. These problems need to be assessed and treated for many functions that these children have the potential to accomplish. It is necessary for physical, occupational, and speech therapists to assess basic visual skills as they relate to motor skills in general, and also to refer the child to an ophthalmologist or developmental optometrist for much needed help in understanding the complex visual issues that are common.

CASE STUDY

To illustrate assessment and treatment planning, here is another case study. This is a 16-year-old boy who has diplegia. He is able to take independent steps across a room and uses Lofstrand® crutches for community mobility. When he was younger, he occasionally used a wheelchair. However, when he outgrew it, he and his family felt that it was not needed because he is capable of walking everywhere he wants to go. His biggest goal right now is to get his driver's license, and he is enrolled at a local rehabilitation center's driver's education program.

As his physical therapist, you ask him if there is still anything he feels he needs to come to therapy for. He states that he has one goal besides his driving, and that is to start using a straight cane more frequently in the community. He feels that he would look better and feel less noticeable to others when he walks. He says that he has tried the cane several times, but has fallen, and that is very embarrassing to him.

Set a short-term (1 month) goal for him to be able to use his cane for at least two evenings per week when he goes somewhere away from home. Have him keep a diary of this. During assessment, you notice that his gait is energy costly due to little or no use of thoracic rota-

tion, poor use of hip abduction during mid-stance, and poor use of plantar flexion in late stance. Because of some bony changes in his hip joints reported by his orthopedist, you believe you probably can affect his thoracic rotation and plantar flexion the most to help make his gait more energy efficient. He has trouble with the cane when he comes to curbs and steps. It is not only that he has difficulty with the necessary weight shifting and strength of lower extremity extension to step up, but he also misjudges height. He has poor development of accurate depth perception. In formally looking at his visual motor control, you note that his eyes do not move together. His right eye is centered well, but his left is usually medially deviated. He has trouble judging some figure-ground tasks (e.g., he cannot see white shoelaces on white tennis shoes and always changes the color of his shoestrings to contrast with his shoes).

Work in therapy first to ensure that he can visually scan, especially with downward gaze, as he moves through space. He is able to move his head and eyes freely, except when he stands and tries to turn to look behind himself. He is afraid to try this because he feels as if he will fall. Work on the ability to do this along with thoracic rotation. Start work on postural holding with the lower trunk while standing, moving his crutches closer to his body as he stands more erect (decreasing his base of support) while you facilitate hip extension. This requires that he first be positioned in slight hip

external rotation, then lean forward toward the front of his base of support while you support his abdominal muscles and lower ribcage to prevent excessive thoracolumbar joint extension. He can do this with, then without, the crutches.

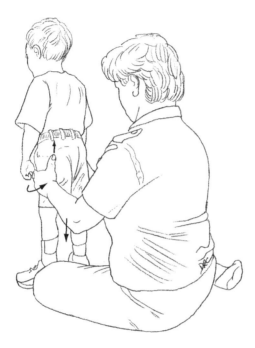

Figure 4.68 After facilitating a more erect posture while moving the crutches closer to himself, this child, who is younger than the one in our case study, is able to stand with his therapist supporting his lower extremities only. His therapist now facilitates hip and knee extension with hip external rotation as he stands. In the teenager, the therapist also would facilitate control on the distal femurs, but would not be able to directly facilitate hip extension on a larger body.

Work on this in standing with feet side by side, then in stride stance in order to add the thoracic rotation. Have the boy practice turning to look over his shoulder from both positions while you hold his lower trunk to help this area of the body with stability. Next work on decreasing support of him in these postures and movements. Practice with the cane. Practice on one

step first, so that he can combine visual scanning, weight shifting with an active trunk, and plantar-flexion strengthening (with hip and knee extension) to rise onto higher and higher steps. Assist him as needed at the lower trunk or over the hip abductors as he shifts weight onto one leg and lifts the other.

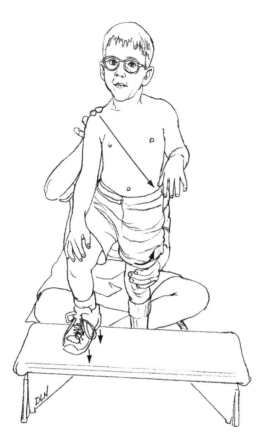

Figure 4.69 As the teenager places one foot on a step, his therapist continues to control the stance leg on the distal femur. She also assists trunk stability by placing one hand over the opposite shoulder and directing pressure towards the stance hip abductor. If his hip abductor could not stabilize his pelvis with this hand placement of the therapist, the therapist would need to change her hand placement to directly support the pelvis laterally.

For his home program, have him practice on a small step with his cane. The entrance to his house would be a good place to do this. He also could keep a diary of when and where he goes using his cane instead of his crutches. He reports later that with practice, he got the *feel* of using the cane and could better judge depth and distance (it may well be that he used sensory systems other than the use of depth perception to help him make the cane be a part of his movement as opposed to the crutches).

Congenital Hemiplegia

Typical Posture and Movement Strategies

Head, neck, tongue, and eyes

The child with hemiplegia truly shows asymmetrical use of the cervical extensor muscles. This is in addition to the asymmetrical head position with which children developing normally, children with quadriplegia, and children with diplegia begin head control. As a result, the child with hemiplegia has two strong factors that lead to very early asymmetrical use of the head—the asymmetrical starting position and a lesion that causes asymmetrical activity between right and left sides of the body. The muscle pull is often stronger on the side with hemiplegia because the lesion typically causes sustained overactivity on that side. As a consequence, the head and eyes are oriented away from the hemiplegic side.

In addition, there are perceptual impairments that orient the head away from the hemiplegic side. Children with hemiplegia may have hemianopsia, a condition in which the visual fields of each eye on the hemiplegic side are impaired. This would mean that for a child with right hemiplegia, the right visual fields in both the left and right eyes are impaired. This provides the child more reason to orient away from the hemiplegic side because visually there is nothing there as far as the child is concerned. In addition, the child also is likely to have a discrepancy in the perception of tactile and proprioceptive information between the two halves of the body. The child is likely to have more accurate perceptual information from the non-hemiplegic side, and so is more likely to orient toward that side.

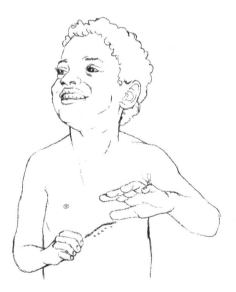

Figure 4.70 This child with left hemiplegia is postured in slight asymmetrical extension of the cervical spine with shortening on the left. He looks to the right and may only be able to look to the right with both eyes.

Children with hemiplegia often are very subtle in their movement compensations. Their asymmetrical head position can be subtle, and the compensations they use to see what is on the hemiplegic side also make the asymmetrical head position less obvious. In order to see what is on the right side of the body, a child with right hemiplegia who has the head shortened by the right cervical extensors with eyes looking to the left simply laterally flexes the head to the left.

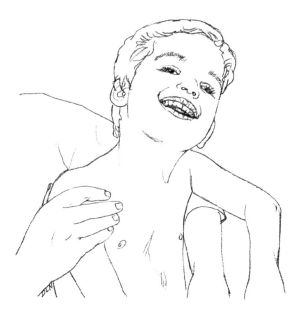

The degree of neck extension and compensatory lateral flexion can vary among children with hemiplegia, but is often subtle. If you watch closely, though, it is likely that the child moves her head using extension and lateral flexion rather than a more mid-position of the head and cervical rotation. Without being able to use rotation, the child's impaired visual fields have less mobility from the orientation of the head. If the child were able to rotate the cervical spine, she could at least have a better ability to visually scan the environment.

Much more subtle than head position may be the mobility and use of the tongue. An assessment of mobility of the tongue for placement for speech sounds and for cleaning food within and outside the mouth may show asymmetry, with the hemiplegic side less mobile.

Functionally, the child with hemiplegia shows early and marked asymmetry of head position that affects visual scanning. This is in addition to other primary impairments of visual field loss that may be present. The disabilities that result prevent full use of visual fields and mobility of the tongue. A 15-month-old is unable to look around the room to see his mother. He cries immediately when she is out of his visual range. Adults interpret this as too strong an attachment to his mother. A 3-year-old is always falling and injuring herself as she runs through the house chasing her siblings. Although the child's parents know that preschoolers fall often when playing, this child has more falls and injuries than her siblings ever did. A 5-year-old eating lunch in her kindergarten class has food on the outside and inside of her mouth that she is not aware of. A teenager cannot get a driver's license because of his visual/perceptual impairments.

Thoracic spine, ribcage, and upper extremities

Children with hemiplegia may show subtle posture and movement compensations in the thoracic spine, but because the upper extremities differ so much from each other, the therapist usually is more aware of problems in this area of the body. Often, the thoracic spine shows asymmetry and mildly increased flexion from lack of development of the relationship between upper extremity use and thoracic extension development. The thoracic spine may follow the head with sustained, overactive extension, which tends to shorten that side of the superficial musculature of the trunk. Because of the increase in muscle contractions on the hemiplegic side, the upper extremity on that side tends to retain and increase shoulder complex elevation with shoulder extension and internal rotation. Elbow flexion, forearm pronation, and a tightly fisted hand follow. This leads to lateral flexion of the spine with concavity on the hemiplegic side, an elevated scapula, and strong holding with superficial trunk muscles, especially the erector spinae and latissimus dorsi. This side of the body does little to no weight bearing through the upper extremity, which often is held away from a surface.

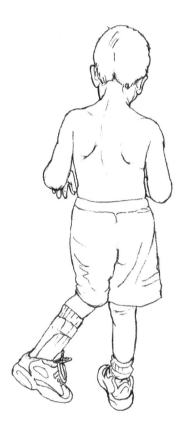

Figure 4.72 This child with hemiplegia shows subtle asymmetries in spine position. His arm on the hemiplegic side is in shoulder complex elevation with shoulder extension. His lower trunk on the left is shortened as is his cervical spine.

The non-hemiplegic upper extremity suffers in its development of control. Because there is lack of full development of thoracic extension and rotation, little to no weight shifting from one weight-bearing arm to the other, and lack of the ability to bring hands together for manual skills, the arm on the non-hemiplegic side may show lack of scapular stability on the ribcage, lack of full use of the rotator cuff muscles in stability of the shoulder joint, lack of graded reach and grasp, and lack of the development of bimanual skills.

Which way does a child with hemiplegia learn to roll when they develop this skill? The answer isn't always immediately clear. But there is a rationale for what they do. Children who develop early sustained cervical and trunk extension with a very stiffly held upper extremity are those who are likely to pull hard with that side of the body to lift themselves up from the surface in prone or supine. They roll over the non-hemiplegic side.

There also are a significant number of children with hemiplegia who are not as stiff and whose sensory-perceptual impairments are more of a problem in their movement than their neuromuscular impairments. Because their sensory losses are so

Congenital Hemiplegia

great on the hemiplegic side and their non-hemiplegic side is more intact, they may learn to push with the more competent non-hemiplegic arm and roll over their hemiplegic side that they cannot feel.

Almost all children with hemiplegia avoid the all-fours position because it demands a certain amount of control, range of motion, and sensory awareness of the hemiplegic arm.

Functionally, the child with hemiplegia has many profound limitations. This child has to use unilateral reaching and manipulation almost exclusively. The child is extremely resistant to learning any function with the hemiplegic arm, for several reasons. First, the other arm works well enough that the child learns to do many things. In addition, this child often is extremely clever in using one arm and the mouth or chin as the other arm, so that toys can be played with. He sees no reason to learn another way. Second, the child's hemiplegic arm is often very impaired in its sensation, so that learning skills with this arm is difficult even if the child is only mildly involved motorically. Third, this child often shows extremes in the perception of tactile information, which is normally used both to discriminate and to protect. Although the child cannot use any of his sensory systems well to discriminate, including the tactile system, he often shows extreme sensitivity in the form of protection. Any tactile message is perceived as a threat, and he pulls away from it. This may be one of the biggest reasons why children with hemiplegia are so difficult to handle physically in treatment.

Disabilities involve the non-use of one arm. A 10-month-old cannot manipulate her toys and has not yet found an efficient way of moving about the floor because she does not assume an all-fours position. She belly crawls, dragging the hemiplegic side of her body as the other side pulls hard to move her forward. A 3-year-old can walk, run, play with many of his toys, feed himself, and scribble with crayons. But he cannot put on or take off a T-shirt, pull up his shorts after toileting, ride his tricycle, use his plastic baseball bat, or swing himself on his swing set. A 7-year-old can walk, run, climb stairs, assist in dressing, and feed himself independently. He falls behind in his schoolwork as he cannot write quickly enough or use the computer with two hands. He also cannot zip and snap his jeans after using the bathroom, and there are some games he cannot play in physical education classes. A 13-year-old goes to a regular middle school and keeps up academically. She walks community distances. She is unable to wash her own hair or style it herself. She needs help with buttons and zippers, and she cannot tie her shoes. She is frustrated in trying to put on make-up that her parents recently told her she could wear.

Lower trunk

The lower trunk often follows the posture of the thoracic area in children with hemiplegia. It shows asymmetry so that the hemiplegic side is shortened, with the pelvis elevated and pulled back. There often is strong contraction and shortening of the erector spinae, latissimus dorsi, and quadratus lumborum that sustains this posture. The lumbar spine is most often in extreme extension, especially in the upper lumbar spine as described in the section on children with diplegia, but with the asymmetry of the lateral flexion added. This places the entire spine in a position that does not enable active rotation, but in a certain degree of passive rotation away from the hemiplegic side (biomechanically the thoracic spine laterally flexes to one side while rotating to the other when the spine is in extension). The extreme extension of the lumbar spine also inhibits use of the abdominal muscles as lower trunk stabilizers.

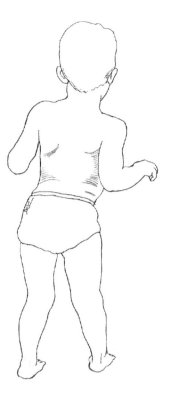

Figure 4.73 This 4-year-old with right hemiplegia shows end range thoracolumbar extension in his posture. He is also shortened on the right side of his trunk as he holds his trunk with the latissimus dorsi and quadratus lumborum muscles. His lower trunk (from about the scapular level down) is rotated slightly to the left. From this position of his lower trunk, his abdominal muscle group is in a lengthened range.

In sitting, the child with hemiplegia has two choices. She can collapse into the lateral flexion of the hemiplegic side so that more weight is taken on that side. This is seen more in children who have less sustained holding of the trunk extensors and who are usually more sensory impaired. The other choice is to elevate the pelvis on the hemiplegic side, hold hard with this elevation, and bear most of the weight on the non-hemiplegic side.

Children with hemiplegia often find a fast, efficient method of moving around the floor before they learn to walk, following all the rules of non-use of the hemiplegic arm and the asymmetry of the spine. In sitting, the child shifts weight onto the non-hemiplegic hip, puts the non-hemiplegic hand on the floor, and scoots about by pushing with the hand and pulling with the leg on the non-hemiplegic side. This is fast and offers a way to avoid all-fours mobility. It also solves the problem of the slowness of belly crawling and rolling while enabling better visual orientation and scanning of the environment.

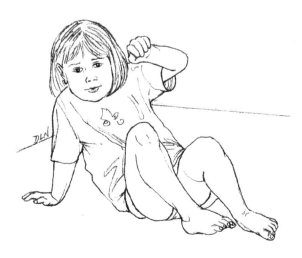

Figure 4.74 This child with left hemiplegia scoots about the floor in this posture. In this way, she can remain in a shortened position in the left side of her trunk and avoid weight bearing through the left extremities. Many children with hemiplegia use this posture to scoot about the floor, totally avoiding an all-fours posture. All fours requires a more symmetrical trunk and certainly more extremity weight bearing than children with hemiplegia are able to use.

Congenital Hemiplegia

Functionally, the child has limitations with the ability to use the lower trunk as an area of controlled stability for the limbs. Because of the abnormal biomechanics and neuro-muscular control, this area of the body does not control the center of mass well. Compensations in other parts of the body substitute for this control. They increase energy expenditure and usually add to the problems of an already poorly aligned body.

The disabilities the child shows can be illustrated as follows. A 16-month-old has learned to sit and scoot about on one hip. She can get in and out of this position from the floor, but has not yet found a way to get up to standing. A 4-year-old can walk, but cannot negotiate stairs without a handrail or stand on one foot while he tries to put on a pair of shorts. A 9-year-old can walk at school and home, but tires at community family outings. She wants to play softball, but is unable to run or swing the bat effectively.

The pelvic girdle and lower extremities

The child with hemiplegia controls the lower extremities several different ways. However, the pelvis is always held asymmetrically in at least two planes. In the coronal plane the pelvis is elevated on the hemiplegic side as previously described. In the transverse plane the pelvis is held so that the hemiplegic side is behind the non-hemiplegic side. Because there are asymmetries in these two planes, it is likely that there are asymmetries in the sagittal plane as well. These asymmetries cause a functional leg length discrepancy with the hemiplegic side seen as shorter because the pelvis is elevated. In addition, there may be a true bony size discrepancy due to growth asymmetries in length and girth.

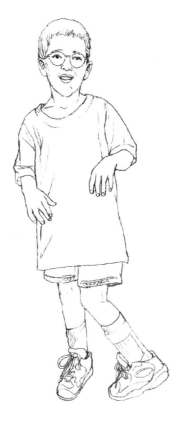

Figure 4.75 This child with hemiplegia uses strong hip internal rotation with slight hip flexion, knee flexion, and plantar flexion. The pelvic elevation on his left side causes the left leg to be shorter functionally. The hip and knee flexion increase its shortness. His plantar flexion, despite the ankle-foot orthosis (AFO), is at least partially a compensation for the short leg–he plantar flexes to reach the ground.

The differences appear in the way the child controls the hip and the rest of the lower extremity from this pelvic position. In children who are very stiff—those who sustain cocontraction with little range of movement in their lower extremity joints—the hip often is held in slight flexion, adduction, and internal rotation. The knee is held in slight flexion with strong cocontraction of the flexors and extensors. The lower leg tends to follow with internal rotation, plantar flexion, and inversion with strong pull of the tibialis posterior. The foot supinates with weight bearing.

The second posture frequently seen in children with hemiplegia is of less hip flexion and internal rotation (although these positions are still present), but including knee hyperextension with weight bearing and plantar flexion, although the heel may appear to touch the floor after the toes contact and the leg is loaded in walking.

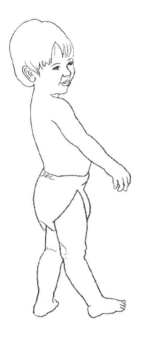

Figure 4.76 This 2-year-old with right hemiplegia stands with lumbar extension, slight hip flexion, knee hyperextension, and plantar flexion. The knee hyperextension is a result of the overactive and tight gastroc-nemius muscles which crosses the knee joint posteriorly. If the child assumed weight on the ball of the foot and did not put the heel down, knee hyperextension would probably not occur.

The third posture is one of slight hip external rotation (or hip internal rotation with the external rotation occurring in the knee joint), a more mobile knee with phases of flexion and extension, and slight plantar flexion with pronation of the foot. This posture is seen in the child who has less neuromuscular stiffness and perhaps more sensory involvement. The leg tends to be dragged behind with the foot seldom leaving the floor during walking.

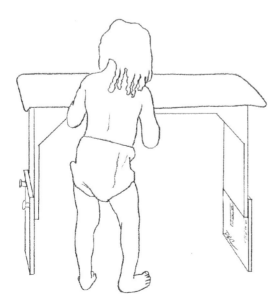

Figure 4.77 This child with right hemiplegia leans her trunk toward the hemiplegic side rather than elevating her pelvis. Her hip and knee are slightly flexed with her hip externally rotated.

Congenital Hemiplegia

Functionally, the child has to contend with at least a functional leg length discrepancy for all walking skills. She also has to contend with asymmetries in control of each lower extremity and with a trunk that does not move fully in all three planes.

Some of the anticipated disabilities are as follows. An 18-month-old who has just learned to walk falls constantly because she drags her right foot on the floor. Therefore, she often refuses to walk and wants to be carried. She cannot get up from the middle of the floor to standing. In her preschool class, she cannot keep up with her peers when they go out to play on the playground—she cannot get on and off any of the equipment designed for toddlers. A 6-year-old can walk, climb stairs with a handrail, step up a curb that is no more than 4 inches high, run, and jump. She cannot step down a curb by herself, ascend or descend stairs without a handrail, or ride her bicycle without training wheels. A 13-year-old experiences low back pain, has scoliosis, and is unable to put his own foot orthotic on or tie his shoes. He also cannot run in physical education class, moving only at a fast walk. He has fallen in the hallway of his middle school several times, and although not seriously hurt, he is very embarrassed.

General Treatment Strategies

Children with hemiplegia are always a challenge to treat because they often can do so much by themselves and see no reason to be interfered with—they reach many of their own functional movement goals. In fact, many children with hemiplegia accomplish a good number of functional skills, but are limited in many others. Almost all children with hemiplegia learn to walk by themselves whether they receive therapy or not. The physical therapist has to anticipate the disabilities the child is likely to have that involve higher-level ambulatory skills. Almost all children with hemiplegia have severe impairments and disabilities involving hand use that must be intensely addressed. And children with hemiplegia run the gamut as far as speech and language needs—some have no disabilities at all, some have mild dysarthria, and some have severe speech, feeding, and cognitive impairments.

Because of the marked asymmetry in neuromuscular control and sensory perception, children with hemiplegia develop a very abnormal perception of their body schema. There is a shift of the sense of midline toward the non-hemiplegic side both motorically and sensorily. Therefore, it takes tremendous work to establish a more correct midline perception of the head and trunk. The limb asymmetry often is obvious, but treating it requires addressing the more subtle asymmetries in the head and trunk. The child must be aligned properly, which means coming out of shortening on the hemiplegic side and out of rotation toward the non-hemiplegic side before beginning any limb movements.

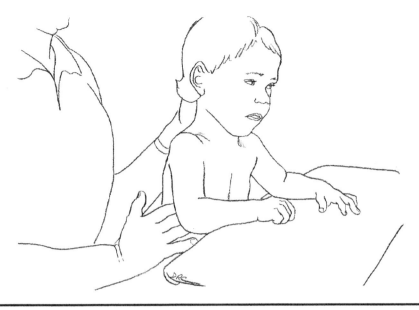

Figure 4.78 In some children with hemiplegia, much work needs to be done to orient vision and head position in symmetry. Here, this child's therapist corrects subtle rotational and lateral flexion asymmetries while facilitating visual gaze in midline. The child will then need to shift his eyes and turn his head from this more symmetrical starting position. Emphasize returning to the starting position frequently to reinforce the motoric and perceptual aspects of posture and movement goals.

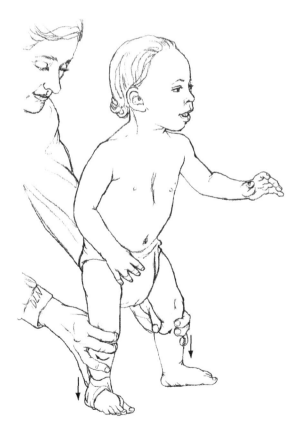

Figure 4.79a Once this toddler's head and trunk position is more symmetrical, her therapist works to help her align both lower legs prior to taking steps. She assists knee extension by giving an external rotation torque to both tibia. As the child's knees extend, the therapist pushes her hands down toward the floor to help the child take her weight through her heels. This provides the child the weight-bearing surface and alignment to become more active with hip, knee, and ankle extension.

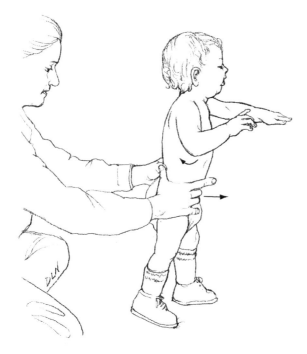

Figure 4.79b Now the therapist helps the child take steps. She supports the child's lower trunk and assists hip extension in the early stance phase of gait. She also assists the slight degree of trunk rotation that accompanies each step (the lower thoracic spine rotates slightly to the right as the child steps through with her left foot).

Active trunk rotation is necessary to both sides in order to achieve smooth reciprocal limb movements and as a basis for limb disassociation.

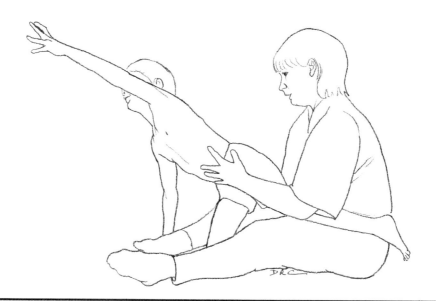

Figure 4.80 This child reaches while his therapist assists active trunk extension with rotation. Trunk rotation is an essential component of active limb disassociation.

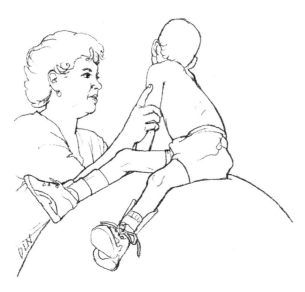

Figure 4.81   Weight bearing on the arms is usually most easily facilitated when the thoracic spine is first assisted to extend and rotate.

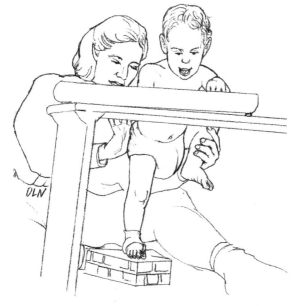

Figure 4.82   This toddler's therapist ensures that her trunk is rotating as she shifts weight onto her hemiplegic lower extremity.

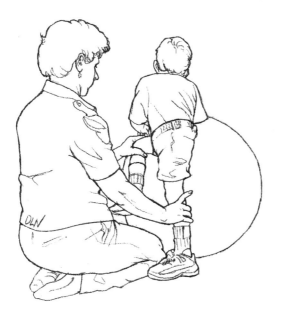

Figure 4.83   This child is able to actively rotate when his therapist asks him to put both hands on the ball. His therapist can then help him move into greater hip extension on his left leg as some of his body weight is supported by the ball.

Both sides of the body must be treated according to their needs. The hemiplegic side needs elongation of shortened muscle and inhibition of muscles holding with sustained contractions in preparation for movement. This side also needs organized, meaningful sensory input starting with firm touch pressure and visual attention to that side to learn new movements.

However, the non-hemiplegic side has needs: Often the scapula on this side, which is needed for controlled placement of the shoulder, is not stable on the ribcage; the trunk does not rotate away from this side; the hip is not well controlled by the abductors and extensors; and the hand doesn't experience bilateral or bimanual activities. Well-graded movements in general are lacking on both sides.

The therapist may ask children with hemiplegia to move to and away from the correct midline in all planes. Specific movements depend entirely on the functional skill that is the child's goal. These often are bilateral skills and involve active use of the non-hemiplegic side to lead and guide the hemiplegic side at first. Transitions to and from the actual midline assist with the integration of both sides of the body.

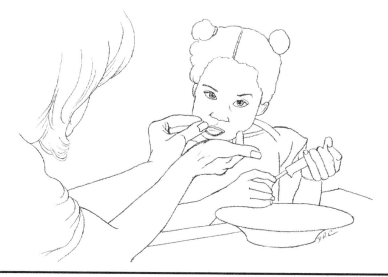

Figure 4.84   This child bites most easily if her head is turned away from her hemiplegic side. Her speech pathologist allows her to begin here, then slowly orients her head toward midline as she repeats biting.

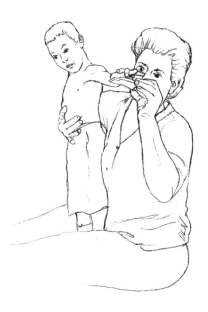

Figure 4.85   This child is reaching with more shoulder abduction and external rotation than he can generate on his own. His therapist assists this primarily through thoracic extension with rotation and support of the alignment of his trunk (so that he doesn't move into excessive lumbar extension). She is less concerned with the type of grasp he uses at this point in his treatment and more concerned with his ability to move his arm away from his body.

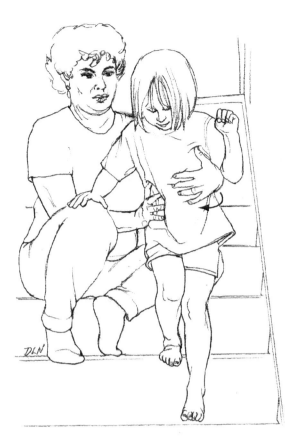

Figure 4.86 This girl with left hemiplegia is learning to descend stairs without upper extremity assist. Her therapist assists trunk rotation toward the midline, then slightly to the right as the child reaches for the step below with her left foot. The therapist then will facilitate movement of the trunk in the opposite direction of rotation when the child reaches for the next step with her right foot.

C A S E   S T U D Y

Look at a 4-year-old child who has left hemiplegia. She is ambulatory. She can walk, run, and climb stairs with a rail. She is able to use her left hand to assist her right for a few skills, such as grasping and holding some toys while she uses her right hand to manipulate and play with them, and she can hold small objects against herself or a tabletop with her left hand. In occupational therapy, it is time to reevaluate her and set new goals. Her grandmother, who is the caretaker, says that she is most concerned about the child's left hand. Even though she also has trouble with her leg, she is able to run and play. The grandmother would like to see the child use her left hand more. The occupational therapist may ask what she envisions the child doing first with that hand if she could use it more. Her grandmother would like her to have the ability to carry some of her bigger toys around, play with the T-ball set she received for her birthday, and hold her cup at the table without spilling it so much. She also

would like to learn to dress and undress herself completely (except for fasteners and shoelaces), but feels that the child is totally uninterested in this and would not cooperate.

The therapist sets a treatment goal for the child to pick up a 6-inch diameter ball from the floor to throw it into a basketball hoop. The child loves to play basketball and can throw the ball into the Little Tikes® hoop quite accurately with her right hand, but cannot pick the ball up from the floor. She rarely turns her head and eyes to the left as she moves through space. She only looks at her left arm with the effort of trying to use it. When this happens, she opens and holds open her mouth as her left arm moves. She also moves extremely slowly with the left arm.

On both formal and informal sensory testing, she shows little ability to move her left arm unless she is looking at it, indicating poor somatosensory awareness. On testing, she did not always cooperate or give selective attention to the testing, but did not indicate any awareness of firm or light touch when she could not see it. More discrete tests such as 2-point discrimination were not only impossible because of lack of attention to the test, but considered well above her capabilities at this point because she did not seem aware of even firm touch. The exception was when her hand was touched or manipulated in any way. She then exhibited a defensive pulling away, along with saying "No!" This may indicate that tactile information is perceived as defensive exclusively in the hand. The therapist also may conclude that the central processing of information from her tactile system may be poorly modulated because she shows both poor awareness in parts of the arm and defensive responses only in her hand.

In treatment, you may decide to start with the basketball activity right away because it is familiar, something she thoroughly enjoys, and a game she will play willingly for as long as someone lets her. You may let her get into difficulty picking the ball up from the floor before intervening physically, so that she will see why you are touching her and helping her hold the ball. You may take hold of both arms firmly and help them move as a unit with shoulder flexion and horizontal adduction with external rotation. Leave her hand alone and try for both arms moving together because it will be harder to gain her trust and acceptance in physically handling her hand. Also, you want her to be immediately successful so that she continues to enjoy the game and understands why you are helping her. Use firm touch to both arms, helping guide the arm or forearm into the desired postures and movements. Use large range, fast movements to give more somatosensory information to her arms. Together, push her hands (the left is in wrist flexion and ulnar deviation with intrinsic muscle tightness) into the ball and make lots of noise with the hands picking up the ball for auditory and somatosensory feedback.

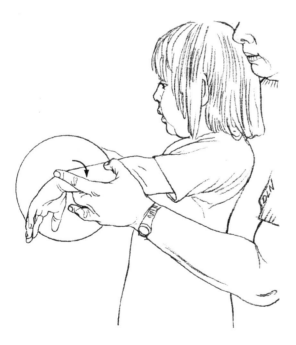

Figure 4.87 This child's therapist helps hold her arms against the ball. She first facilitates shoulder flexion with horizontal adduction so that the child is successful in holding the ball and so that the child enjoys the game. The therapist will next work to roll the shoulder into external rotation and the forearm out of pronation toward a more neutral position.

Begin to facilitate a more symmetrical trunk by giving traction to her left arm when lifting it overhead with shoulder flexion and external rotation. Because of mild asymmetries of posture in the trunk, assist movement of the trunk to the right, back to midline, to the left, and back to midline. As her trunk is better aligned and as she works through input to her somatosensory systems, the voluntary stiffness of her left upper extremity decreases. Her hand more automatically opens then. At this point, support her wrist in extension and slight radial deviation. She easily opens and closes her left hand on the ball, and although her fingers are still poorly aligned with no use of hand intrinsics, she is doing much more than she was thirty minutes ago. It is more important to end the session with many positive changes in simple patterns of functional hand opening and closing while having fun, than it is to make her try more physically challenging skills that are very difficult for her. As rapport builds, challenge her in ways that can be sensorially uncomfortable and/or motorically more difficult.

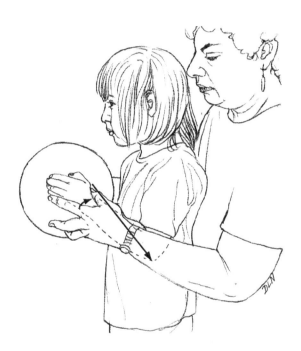

Figure 4.88 After the therapist engages the child in an enjoyable game, she begins to handle the hand, the area of this child's body where she most resists touch. The therapist radially deviates and extends her wrist, followed by giving direction to the pressure toward the child's elbow. The child is able to contact the ball with the heel of her hand and her fingertips, but she does not yet have enough muscle length in her long finger flexors to contact the ball with the entire palmar surface of her hand.

For her home program, ask her grandmother to play one game with her a day that involves both arms holding or carrying something large (but not too heavy). Show her grandmother how to hold both arms at the same time and *wiggle* them rapidly and firmly just prior to asking the child to hold or carry the object. Explain that she will work on better hand posture and function with time, but that this is an extremely important first step. Emphasize that the child must be pushed to learn to do new skills with her hand, but also respect the sensations she gets in her hand when it is touched.

Children With Athetosis

Pathophysiology

Children with athetosis (from the Greek *athetos*, meaning not stationary) probably have damage to the basal ganglia, mainly due to perinatal asphyxia or severe jaundice (Yokochi, Shimabukuro, Kodama, Kodama, & Hosoe, 1993). The putamen, which is part of the basal ganglia, shows damage on MRI scans in some infants with athetosis (Foley, 1992; Rutherford, Pennock, Murdoch-Eaton, Cowan, & Dubowitz, 1992). The basal ganglia are particularly vulnerable to hypoxia. The thalamus also seems to be damaged in some children with athetoid cerebral palsy. The majority are born full term, although these babies often have low birth weight, suggesting that lesions may occur during pregnancy from chronic hypoxia rather than from traumatic birth events (Foley, 1992). The birth asphyxia may be an expression of problems that already exist. Hagberg and Hagberg (1992) are not convinced that we yet know which causes what—does birth asphyxia cause athetosis or do prenatal events cause the difficult birth? There are many research questions as yet unanswered.

The basal ganglia are a set of interconnected structures in the forebrain (Rosenbaum, 1991). They regulate the postural background interplay of flexors and extensors for voluntary movement as well as the timing of movements and the intensity of muscle contractions. Other areas of the brain also regulate this interplay, including the cerebral cortex, cerebellar pathway, and brainstem pathway. The basal ganglia are also part of the motor-planning system, sending sensory information to the pre-motor cortex, and seem to play a role in initiating movement sequences.

Athetosis in cerebral palsy is less common than hypertonia. However, there are a significant number of children who have both hypertonia and athetosis because of more diffuse damage of the CNS. Also, athetosis as a diagnosis is subject to widely differing interpretation based on physicians' and therapists' exposure to and understanding of this type of cerebral palsy. One reason is that there is not a common language used by the medical professions in identifying and describing athetosis. To many people the term is used to describe a child with writhing limb movements that are rather quick and change rapidly between flexion and extension. To others the child with athetosis can show many other characteristics in movement control that are described later. Indeed, there are children with athetosis who do not present the picture of a constantly moving, writhing child. Because athetosis may include damage to different parts of the basal ganglia and thalamus, the lesion in one child will be different than the lesion in the next, so that differing movement problems may emerge.

In describing the pathophysiologies possible in children with athetosis, it helps to start with definitions of terms. The problem is that many authors use these terms differently, so that more confusion arises; in most of the research literature, the terms are used but not defined. In addition, the dictionary offers only generalized descriptions, many of which seem extremely similar. In reality, we probably are using different words to mean the same thing in describing children with athetosis; these commonly used terms really do not describe the range of impairments, functional limitations, and disabilities.

> **Athetosis:** A condition in which there is a constant succession of slow, writhing, involuntary movements of flexion and extension, pronation and supination of the fingers and hands, and sometimes of the toes and feet. Usually caused by an extrapyramidal lesion (Stedman's Medical Dictionary [Stedman's], 1995).

> **Chorea:** Irregular, spasmodic, involuntary movements of the limbs or facial muscles, often accompanied by hypotonia (Stedman's, 1995). A ceaseless occurrence of a wide variety of rapid, highly complex, jerky, dyskinetic movements that appear to be well coordinated but are performed involuntarily (Dorland's Illustrated Medical Dictionary [Dorland's], 1994).

> **Choreoathetosis:** A combination of chorea and athetosis.

> **Dystonia:** A state of abnormal tonicity in any of the tissues (Stedman's, 1995). Dyskinetic movements due to disordered tonicity of muscle (Dorland's, 1994).

> **Dyskinesia:** Distortion or impairment of voluntary movement (Dorland's, 1994). Difficulty in performing voluntary movements. Term usually used in relation to various extrapyramidal disorders (Stedman's, 1995).

The terms that are used most to describe children with athetosis are very close in meaning and difficult to distinguish from each other. All describe a disorder of voluntary control with involuntary, complex movements present. Although it often is true that children with athetosis show highly complex, uncontrolled, and seemingly involuntary movements, this does not help the therapist see the whole picture; possible impairments in the different systems that contribute to movement control; or the reasons for the similarities in posture and movement control often seen among a wide variety of children and adults with athetosis.

The purpose of this chapter is to describe these children in more detail, offering possible explanations to help the therapist clinically understand the impairments and functional limitations. The following description of the impairments, posture and movement strategies, functional limitations, and disabilities focus on a child who has athetosis without any hypertonicity. This is for the purpose of sorting out impairments caused by a particular area of lesions. Some children will more closely fit the picture described and are more *pure* in their athetosis than others. There are many more children who have characteristics described in this chapter as well as characteristics of hypertonicity described in Chapter 4.

As a therapist, there are advantages to being able to sort out the impairments. Treatment will be more exact and directed at managing movements in the individual child. For example, a child may be very floppy at rest, assuming wide-based, asymmetrical postures that serve as the alignment from which he initiates movement. However, when he starts to move, he immediately becomes very stiff with excessive use of cocontraction and limited ranges of movement, and then holds this position. Suddenly, this cocontraction ceases and he cannot generate any muscle activity at all for a few seconds. He assumes a position of passive total flexion, whereas a second ago he was stiffly in total extension. This would suggest that there may be impairments both from hypertonicity and athetosis. Understanding that you must manage both excessive cocontraction and then no contraction at all a few seconds later changes your treatment techniques and sequences.

A related advantage is that you are prepared to watch for changes in the presentation of impairments over time. There are many children who, in the first months or years of their lives, present with hypertonicity. Once some of the resulting impairments are successfully managed, you may begin to see more subtle impairments that were masked by the strong influence of hypertonicity. The athetoid component of the child's CP may be emerging. For example, I have seen several children who were very stiff as infants with classic signs of spasticity and hypertonicity. Once they began moving more successfully and their CNS continued to mature, other signs emerged, such as rapid alternating flexion and extension of the fingers, more asymmetrical posturing, large-range sagittal plane movements of the tongue between protrusion and retraction, and postures with more end-range positions. On the other hand, I have seen severely involved children who were hypotonic for several years with classic postures associated with hypotonicity begin to show the impairments seen in athetosis once they finally achieved any degree of movement against gravity. As a therapist, it is wise to continually observe and assess so as to be prepared for what may happen next.

Another reason for careful observation over time is that, as a team member who is likely to see the child more frequently than others on the team, you may have information that is valuable for the rest. Certain surgeries, medications, orthotics, and equipment tend to be designed for and work best for specific impairments. A surgeon who sees the child once or twice in the office may not have seen the impairments that may make the surgery less successful, or even inadvisable. The neurologist considering a medication for the management of spasticity needs information on other impairments the child shows that may interfere with the intended action of the drug. An orthotic that works well managing a poorly aligned ankle in a child with moderate hypertonicity may be poorly tolerated by a child with athetosis, even if it helps the alignment. Discussing as much information as possible with other team members helps them make better decisions about treatment choices, just as their information helps you make better decisions.

Impairments in Athetoid Cerebral Palsy

Neuromuscular system
Reflexive tone

The child with pure athetosis is likely to show depressed deep tendon reflexes.

Difficulty with muscle contraction

Children with athetosis have differing problems in control of starting and stopping muscle contractions. Common problems include poor ability to initiate movement because the antagonist is overactive, poor ability to initiate and terminate activity because of excessive contraction that tends to increase with effort, and initiation of the antagonist rather than the intended agonist. Some children with athetosis sustain muscle activity too much, whereas others cannot sustain it sufficiently to complete a task. It also may be true that some children sustain too much in some areas of the body and not enough in others, or that at different times the child sustains sufficiently, too much, or too little. Because the pathophysiology is assumed to be in the basal ganglia in children with athetosis, it makes sense that timing and initiation of movements are abnormal.

Grading agonist/antagonist activity

In children with athetosis, there is extreme variability when using movements that require the interaction of antagonists. Many describe the movements in athetosis as involuntary and leave the description at that. Although unpredictable force and initiation of movement with the opposite muscle group of that required for the intended movement often occur, there frequently is some consistency to these movements. Each child's postures and movements are often typical of that child, and so I question the *involuntary* part that is so widely attributed to athetosis.

Hallett and Alvarez (1983) agree. In their research of reaching patterns in adults with athetoid CP, they noted that the spontaneous activity of their patients suggests that many of the involuntary movements are inappropriate and excessive activity brought about by voluntary movements. Their research involved 14 adults whose rapid elbow movements were recorded on EMG. The normal reaction on EMG to rapid, ballistic movements is a triphasic burst of activity, first from the agonist, then the antagonist, and then the agonist again. This requires a reciprocal interaction of flexors and extensors. In Hallett and Alvarez's subjects with athetosis, six distinct patterns were seen on EMG with the voluntary effort of rapid elbow flexion. This suggests that not all athetosis is alike—the way one person controls the effort of a rapid movement may be quite unlike the next person. Although each subject had characteristic patterns of movement, some showed more than one pattern when attempting the same reaching task.

Other literature provides reports of general abnormal cocontraction patterns, *contrary* movements in which the antagonist contracts instead of the agonist, and alternations between flexion and extension in movement efforts in posture (Foley, 1983; Hadders-Algra, Bos, Martijn, & Prechtl, 1994; Yokochi, et al., 1993). Remember that Hallett and Alvarez were looking at more ballistic (feedforward) movements, whereas other literature may look more at postural control that enables sensory feedback in the system's final decision about control.

As a clinician, it is imperative to take the time to figure out how each child with athetosis moves. Some children may use more cocontraction with effort, which seems to make their movements less functional. Others may *wind up* to move, extending before flexing, but are eventually able to accomplish the task. Others may need to quiet the overactivity of the antagonist before beginning to move. Understanding such variability is difficult and time consuming, but necessary if the effects of therapy are to make movements more predictable and functional for the child.

Limited synergies used to produce posture and movement

In addition to the problems noted by Hallett and Alvarez (1983), Nashner et. al. (1983) showed that postural reactions were abnormal in a child with athetosis just as ballistic movements are. In this study, only one subject had athetosis. The response to disturbed balance was similar to that seen in the subjects with hypertonicity. The proximal muscles of the lower body tended to fire first, and there was variability in the relationship between the synergists in contraction time. This ordering of muscle activity is the reverse of that seen in people without disability, who fire distal muscles prior to proximal in the lower body and who time muscle contractions of synergists precisely to stabilize the body when balance is disturbed.

Sensory/Perceptual systems

Children with athetosis seem less likely to have primary impairments of eye muscle imbalance than children with hypertonicity (Foley, 1983) and may be more able to control eye movements for communication than can children with other types of cerebral palsy. However, there are impairments of the eyes in some children with athetosis. Nystagmus may be present as well as problems with pursuit movements. Upward visual gaze has been viewed as a primary impairment (Foley, 1983), but also may be a secondary impairment similar to the way that other children with CP use the upward gaze to assist head lifting. Because children with athetosis tend to assume and use extremely asymmetrical postures (see section on *typical posture and movement strategies* on page 152), the upward visual gaze often is in the extreme peripheries of the eyes.

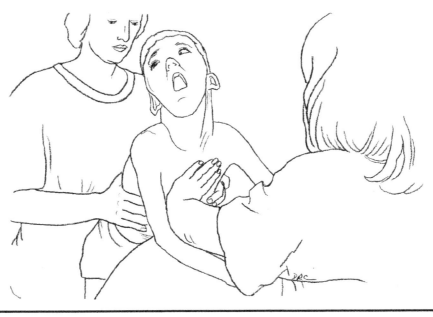

Figure 5.1 This 10-year-old with athetosis assists head lifting with cervical, jaw, and eye extension. Since he lifts from an asymmetrical starting position, his eyes not only extend (upward gaze), but are in the upper right visual fields.

One area of complexity in the vision of children with athetosis is the way they control the head and eyes in order to move. In some of the literature, children with athetosis are described as using gaze aversion when attempting reaching or other motor skills. This is seen as a primary impairment of an absent or abnormal ocular reflex. While this may be true to some extent, looking away from what the child is reaching for may have a more thorough explanation that is described in *typical posture and movement strategies* on page 152. Looking away while reaching is part of an entire synergy used in an effort to gain postural stability. It can be influenced and changed to a certain extent in almost all children with athetosis and must be influenced for the teaching of many functional skills.

Research has shown that children with athetosis have a less than normal kinesthetic sense (sense of movement and position), but not to the degree that children with hypertonicity have (Opila-Lehman, Short, & Trombly, 1985). Clinically, many children with athetosis learn well from kinesthetic information provided actively during therapy and with repetition. They often can remember and use information about position and movement gradation after being shown how a movement should be performed, paired with appropriate verbal and visual cues. Therapists often rely on this in teaching more functional movement because children with athetosis seem to have more intact perceptual skills than motor execution skills.

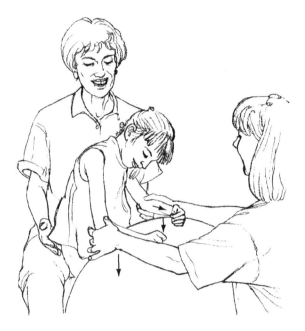

Figure 5.2   This girl's therapists use firm pressure of her forearms into the therapy ball. The purpose of this is to help her actively move her head into the midline and to bring her eyes out of upward gaze.

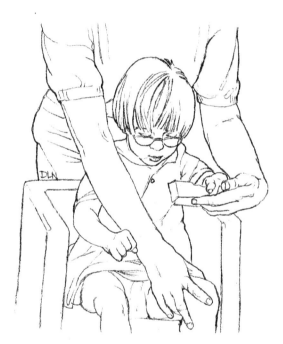

Figure 5.3   This child is guided visually, tactilely, and proprioceptively into a more midline position of her head and trunk before she reaches for her toy.

It has been suggested that children with athetosis have a very strong and repetitive response to tactile information. It is not so much that they are tactilely defensive; rather, they are tactilely overresponsive. Any tactile information causes a prolonged and repetitive response of exaggerated movement, increased movement frequency, or both. If this theory is correct, it may help explain several clinical observations. Children with athetosis often are opposed to bracing, splinting, and wheelchair designs that provide intermittent skin contact as they move inside or against it. They tend to pull away after contact with the equipment and often refuse to use it. Perhaps tactile sensitivity is at least part of the reason. Children with athetosis also respond favorably to the use of Lycra® splinting that comes in firm contact with the skin and is designed to allow movement while supporting joints (Blair, Ballantyne, Horsman, & Chauvel, 1995; Chauvel, Horsman, Ballantyne, & Blair, 1993). The

Chapter Five

response of some children with athetosis wearing these specially designed garments has been an increase in hand function, a decrease in involuntary movements, and a more stable head and trunk, sometimes with less asymmetry. Although the explanations for these observations are still to be determined, one hypothesis may be that they reduce the tactile information that causes such hyperresponsiveness. Or, it may be that they provide deep pressure into the proprioceptive system, which could have an organizing effect.

Another clinical observation goes along with the Lycra splinting use. Some children with athetosis function better with less extraneous movement when they wear tight clothing such as bicycle shorts and leotards. This observation comes from therapists who have suggested the idea to families or families who discovered it on their own. Also, in children who need head supports on their wheelchairs and who move their heads excessively, sometimes wearing a sweatband type of headband where the head tends to rub the head support helps reduce the unwanted head movements.

Children who have athetosis caused by jaundice are susceptible to hearing loss. Although this has been seen as a decreasing cause of athetosis over the years because of better neonatal management, there has been an alarming increase in undetected jaundice in newborns who are sent home 24 hours after birth. If this practice remains unchanged, there may be an increase in impairments because of the effects of jaundice.

Children with athetosis also may be very responsive to sudden or loud noises, similar to children with hypertonicity. Many times the response to sound is a sudden loss of any postural control the child had or a sudden change in position along with eye widening, indicating distress.

Musculoskeletal system

Children with athetosis are likely to develop fewer contractures than children with hypertonia, but the ones they develop often are severe. Because they move more frequently and through larger ranges than children with hypertonicity, the likelihood of the secondary impairments of many joint contractures decreases. However, because many children with athetosis use only a few postures and movements rather than a wide variety, contractures can develop in ranges where muscles are not able to move joints. In addition, children with athetosis use strong, repetitive postures to try to control themselves against gravity, as described in *typical posture and movement strategies* on page 152. These postures also tend to shorten muscles and deform bones and joints. Muscles that tend to shorten include the pectorals, upper cervical extensors, latissimus dorsi, scapular elevators, rectus abdominus, intercostals, forearm pronators, wrist and finger flexors, thumb extensors and abductors, hamstrings, ankle dorsiflexors, ankle evertors, and toe flexors. Shortness tends to be severe in these muscles.

Children with athetosis also develop common areas of excessive mobility or overlengthened musculature which, therefore, are secondary impairments. Because of repetitive, exaggerated postures and movements, the child with athetosis is susceptible to these impairments. Those commonly seen are:

- instability of the jaw with temporomandibular joint (TMJ) deformity possible

- overlengthening of the infrahyoid muscles

- instability of the cervical spine (described in detail on page 148)

- instability or dislocation of the shoulder joint in any direction, but often inferiorly

- hyperextension at the elbow

- hyperextension of the interphalangeal joints of the fingers and thumb

- overlengthening of the anterior hip capsule and ligaments

- overlengthening of the plantar flexors and ankle invertors

Other serious secondary impairments that develop from not only the typically assumed postures but from the strong pushing into these postures are:

- **Hip dislocation.** It is not uncommon to see a teenager or adult with athetosis develop an anterior dislocation of one hip. This often is due to a pushing of the lumbar spine and hips into extension, often from a supine or sitting position, an extremely asymmetrical starting position. It takes time to dislocate a hip anteriorly because of the strong ligaments and joint capsule anteriorly, but with repetitive pushing of the hips into extension, it can be done. With a posteriorly dislocated hip, it is hard to extend and abduct the hip for standing. Also, this leg becomes functionally shorter. With an anteriorly dislocated hip, it is difficult to flex the hip, which makes assuming the sitting position difficult, if not impossible. People with spastic athetosis may dislocate one hip anteriorly and one posteriorly (see Chapter 4 for a description of the probable mechanisms of posterior hip dislocation).

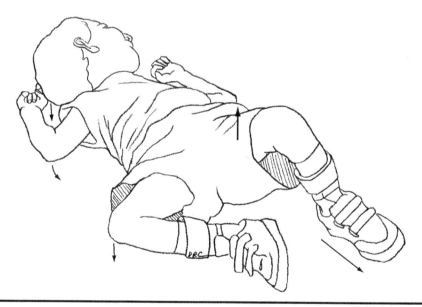

Figure 5.4 This 5-year-old with severe hypotonia and athetosis is pushing himself back in supine. As he lifts his hips up from the surface using extension in his cervical and lumbar spine from an asymmetrical starting position, he places stretch on the anterior hip joint. If he repeats this movement over years, especially if his extension becomes stronger and more asymmetrical, he could eventually anteriorly dislocate one or both hips.

- **Cervical spine instability.** A life-threatening secondary impairment that can develop is malalignment, narrowing of the spinal canal, spondylosis, and radiculomyelopathy of the cervical spine as a result of excessive and/or abnormal movement of the head over years (Fuji et. al., 1987; Harada et al., 1996; Reese, Msall, Owen, Pictor, & Paroski, 1991). This usually is not seen until the adult years. These impairments can cause quadriplegic paralysis, muscular weakness, loss of bowel and bladder control, and loss of functional skills. Any instability of the cervical spine can be life threatening. The treatment is almost always surgical. There are, of course, complications in trying to stabilize the cervical spine with internal fixation in people with athetosis—because the movement disorder is severe with exaggerated, often changing postures and movements, the stability of the internal fixation can be threatened.

- **Thoracic kyphosis and scoliosis.** Although kyphosis tends to be increased in the thoracic area of the spine in most children with any type of cerebral palsy, it is in children with athetosis that we usually see a severely increased kyphosis. This probably develops as a compensatory posture to the child's strong cervical and lumbar/hip extension. It develops to bring the center of mass back over the base of support in sitting and standing, to counterbalance the extension in the cervical and lumbar spine that tends to knock the child over backward. The child uses the strong, tight pectorals and latissimus muscles to help internally rotate the elevated shoulder girdle and to bring the thoracic spine into flexion.

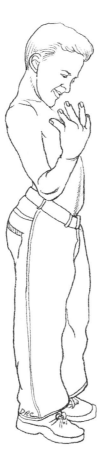

Figure 5.5 This 13-year-old with athetosis stands with strong end range lumbar extension and a thoracic kyphosis. He sustains his head in an active chin tuck to further ensure that his lumbar extension does not knock him over backward. His hand appears very large in this drawing because his elbow is held tightly at his side, his shoulder is slightly externally rotated, and his wrist is flexed (the hand is coming straight at the camera in the photo from which this picture is taken).

The development of scoliosis may be related to both the open-packed, unstable position of the thoracic spine and to the severe asymmetry of postures and movements that children with athetosis assume. See Chapter 4 for a more detailed description of the development of scoliosis.

- **A shift of the hyoid bone and laryngeal system.** Because of the pushing of the cervical spine into strong extension, usually with asymmetry, the anterior surface of the neck overlengthens. This causes the head to be positioned in extreme extension, especially the head on the cervical spine. The masseter muscle also may overlengthen. The hyoid and laryngeal system stay elevated and tipped forward anteriorly. The tongue and laryngeal system are not stabilized posteriorly with muscle activity, as the muscles are so poorly aligned. The child may push the tongue against the palate to attempt stability, which compromises its function for phonation and swallowing (Owens, personal communication, 1998).

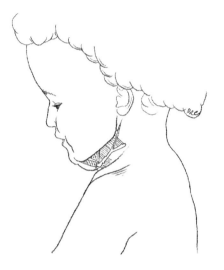

Figure 5.6a This is the normal position of the suprahyoid muscles, hyoid bone, and larynx in an 8-month-old child.

Adult with athetosis   Adult without disability

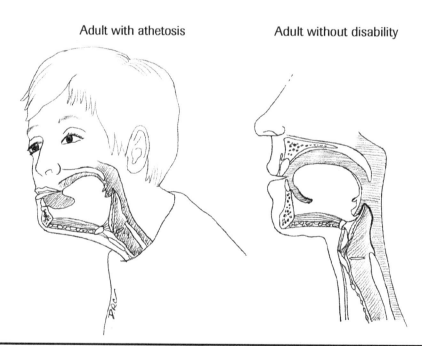

Figure 5.6b Compare the normal child in Figure 5.6a to the normal adult structure in Figure 5.6b on the right. Then compare both of these to the adult with athetosis pictured (Figure 5.6b, left). The person with athetosis shows overstretching of the anterior neck, overstretching of the posterior soft tissues that support the hyoid bone, and a more infant-like position of the hyoid bone. Her tongue is elevated posteriorly to the palate for stability. Correcting this person's alignment out of asymmetrical cervical extension to symmetry and flexion of the head on the cervical spine could greatly interfere with her ability to breathe. The more normal alignment may block her airway with the tongue so retracted and the muscular support of her airway so malaligned.

The child with athetosis develops secondary impairments of lack of strength throughout the full ranges of all joints. As in children with hypertonia, this may be more of a secondary impairment due to lack of use, lack of the ability to sustain muscle activity, and poor alignment for the development of muscular tension. Perhaps strength cannot develop fully because of nutritional factors. It is estimated that adults with athetosis have increased energy requirements due to the uncontrolled, extraneous movements they make, resulting in an average increase of the resting metabolic rate of 524 kcal/day (Johnson, Goran, Ferrara, & Poehlman, 1996). This, combined with the difficulty in grading jaw movements for feeding and the poor ability of the surface of the tongue to provide precision for eating—the base of the tongue is poorly stabilized—may add to the difficulty in taking in the calories needed to build muscle bulk.

On the other hand, children with athetosis may develop adequate strength in portions of the muscles used frequently and repetitively. These usually are those that work in shortened ranges. For example, children with athetosis use their pectorals to assist the thoracic spine into flexion to balance the strong cervical and lumbar/hip extension. The muscles become very tight and very strong in this shortened range.

Another example is the use of the hamstrings distally. Children with athetosis often use the hamstrings to flex the knees in standing and to help hold themselves up in sitting. This is to counterbalance the powerful extension and help prevent them from falling backward. The medial hamstrings may be able to sustain muscle activity in very shortened ranges for this function and, therefore, become quite strong.

Respiratory system

Children with athetosis have a great deal of difficulty coordinating breathing with the onset of voicing and with swallowing. They show bursts of phonatory activity, if they are able to produce sounds, just as the rest of their body shows bursts of muscular activity. Respiration often is arrhythmical, and there is great difficulty controlling exhalation with voicing. They may attempt to voice at the end of their exhalation. It is not uncommon to see children with athetosis who have normal intelligence have the inability to produce sounds because these impairments are so severe. These are children who benefit from learning to communicate through augmentative communication systems. Their language base is adequate for this type of communication, eye movements often are preserved well enough that eye pointing is a possibility to access the system, or they may be able to use one hand or the head with enough control to access the system.

The secondary impairments that develop regarding alignment of the hyoid bone and the laryngeal system must be taken seriously. You must pay careful attention to the child's ability to breathe and swallow if you decide to try to begin to correct alignment for eating or voicing. Quickly placing the person (especially older children and adults who have had time to develop the malalignment) in normal alignment can totally block respiratory efforts and must be avoided. Slowly moving toward better alignment with constant assessment of breathing status is your job as a therapist. Some older children and adults may not be able to breathe with the head position totally corrected, but with treatment may be able to eat and voice with less asymmetry than previously. If their head is in a more midline position, they have the opportunity to better visualize the food or to see to whom they are speaking.

Typical Posture and Movement Strategies
Head, neck, tongue, and eyes

The child with pure athetosis often can be a full-term baby. But because of the patho-physiology that caused the impairments, this child is extremely hypotonic at first, pre-sumably from some hypoxic-ischaemic episode(s). The appearance of the typical bursts of movement, extraneous movement, and alternations between flexion and extension, which are the clinical signs of athetosis, may not be seen for months and usually are not seen until at least after the first year of life (Rutherford et al., 1992). Some children who develop athetosis stay clinically hypotonic for many months, well past the first or second year. They do not show the bursts of extension from an asym-metrical position, as well as the other typical neuromuscular impairments, for quite some time and develop their movement strategies until that time in ways that are sim-ilar to children with severe hypotonia. Perhaps this happens because their impair-ments are severe enough that almost all movement is impossible to generate.

The child with athetosis learns to lift and hold his head up, if he can do it at all, from an extremely asymmetrical base. Remember that children with hypertonia and mild to moderate hypotonia do so too, but their asymmetry is not as great. If you think about a child lying prone who has no disability, the cheek usually rests against the surface. A child with hypertonia may lie the same way or perhaps more on the side of the face with a little more asymmetry. However, the child with severe hypoto-nia who may later develop athetosis rests her weight on the ears. The large, heavy occiput is pulled into gravity with no muscular resistance. This is the starting point from which the child with athetosis tries to learn to lift and hold the head up.

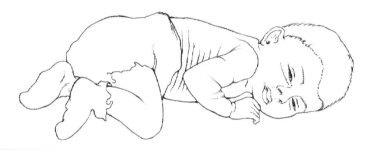

Figure 5.7 This newborn lies prone with hips flexed and her head and spine asym-metrically positioned. Her weight is on the cheek of her face.

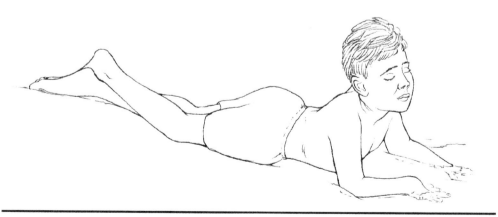

Figure 5.8 This 8-year-old with hyper-tonia lying prone at the water's edge on the beach lifts and holds his head up with slightly asymmetrical extension.

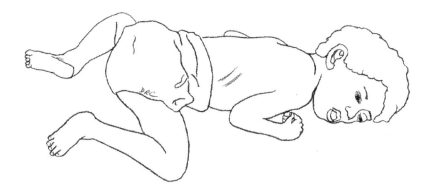

Figure 5.9   This young child is severely hypotonic. There is little to no activity in the postural trunk muscles. The limbs rest against the support surface and are very inactive. The child may pull a little with the hip flexors. His arms will take no weight nor push against the surface and his legs remain extremely abducted. His head is rotated completely to one side. If he does begin to lift his head (and this has taken years for some children), he will initiate the extension from a very asymmetrically positioned head. This sets up the strong asymmetry seen in children with athetosis.

The child may lie like this for months if placed in prone or lie with just as much asymmetry in supine. If placed in an infant seat, the strong asymmetry will still be marked, as the child falls into gravity. Once the child can begin to move, the impairments of athetosis cause him to be able to generate only quick, usually forceful, unsustained movements. Because extension usually is used first in all babies, the child with athetosis may learn first to use these quick bursts of extension in all positions. The extension may be so forceful that the cervical spine and lumbar spine extend simultaneously, causing a strong arching of the spine.

The cervical flexors are quickly and forcefully overlengthened with strong, asymmetrical cervical extension, especially the infrahyoids, and the malalignment of the hyoid and laryngeal system begins. This overlengthening may be asymmetrical, as the child with athetosis may lift the head with it rotated to one side only.

The eyes follow or lead the head movement. Because the head starts from such an asymmetrical position, the eyes are used in the peripheries. Upward gaze (eye extension) often is used to lead and assist head movement. It seems to help the child hold the head up longer and more predictably. And because this strategy may be so successful, the child may learn to use eye extension to lead any body movement. Of course, this means that the eyes are not available for the use they were intended—to seek and scan for information to learn, make social contact, and to help control a variety of postures and movements.

Jaw extension (mouth opening) can and often is part of this overall, forceful extension used to try to control the head. The jaw opening is forceful, and completed through full range. It often sustains in this open position and cannot release until the child drops the head. But because the jaw extension is performed with a very asymmetrical head position, the jaw opens asymmetrically too, enabling abnormal lateral movements to begin at the TMJs. Part of the facial *grimacing* seen in children with athetosis may originate with this asymmetrical, forceful jaw opening.

Children With Athetosis

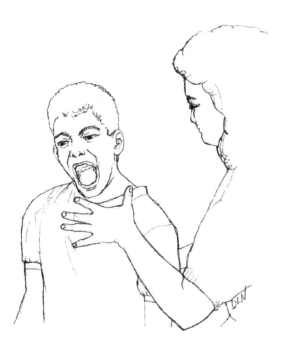

Figure 5.10 This teenager forcefully opens his mouth with his head asymmetrically positioned.

The child with athetosis uses strong tongue retraction, perhaps in an attempt to assist head extension as well as to hold the head against gravity. The suprahyoid muscles are normally tight at birth, and babies typically use tongue retraction when they cry and with efforts to move antigravity. Perhaps the child with athetosis does the same thing, only with more forcefulness and with more frequency. Clinically, it appears that the tongue protrusion often seen in children with athetosis is the way that the child tries to clear the tongue for swallowing and breathing. As is typical for children with athetosis, this protrusion is forceful and extreme in range. In other words, the tongue protrusion is not the original problem, but a solution to moving the strongly retracted tongue. If this is so, the therapist must deal with the problem of tongue retraction to treat the problem of tongue protrusion.

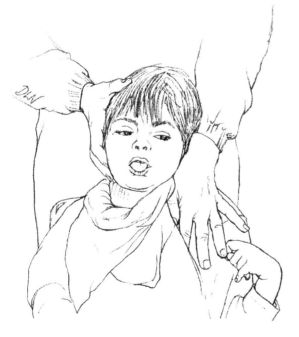

Figure 5.11 This child forcefully protrudes her tongue. She may only have sagittal plane movements available for tongue movements just as she has sagittal plane movements available for the rest of her body. To facilitate more midrange movements of the tongue, her therapist must help her initially position her tongue out of retraction, then assist active movements.

Some children with athetosis learn to use forceful cervical flexion to hold the head up or to counterbalance the tendency for strong extension. This flexion is performed with the large cervical flexors, resulting in a mass flexion without midrange control of the head on the neck. This flexion can be the primary way a child with athetosis holds her head, or it may be a choice that some children can develop for certain postures or movements, including attempts to move prone to W-sitting; to stabilize vision; in speaking; and to stand.

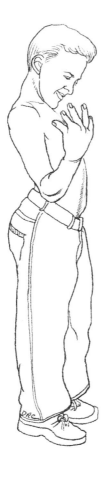

Figure 5.12   This 13-year-old with athetosis stands with strong end range lumbar extension and a thoracic kyphosis. He sustains his head in an active chin tuck to further ensure that his lumbar extension does not knock him over backward. His hand appears very large in this drawing because his elbow is held tightly at his side, his shoulder is slightly externally rotated, and his wrist is flexed.

Functionally, limitations arise from the severe asymmetry of the head, the forceful extension initially used to attempt head control, and the accompanying tongue, jaw, and eye movements to assist that extension. Forceful cervical flexion also may interfere with attaining functional skills in some children.

The disabilities that typically result from movement compensations in this area are as follows: a 10-month-old cannot suck on the bottle well enough to get adequate nutrition, thereby necessitating alternate feeding strategies or more frequent and extremely time-consuming feedings from her caregivers. A 3-year-old cannot move about on the floor at all, but can communicate with yes and no responses using his eyes when placed in adaptive seating. A 5-year-old can scoot on the floor in supine only, cannot sit alone, and eats only pureed food fed by her mother. A 10-year-old is able to sit when placed in a regular chair, but would fall off if left unattended. He can move about the floor on his knees in a sort of bunny-hopping manner, but has no other unassisted mobility. However, he can access a computer and augmentative communication device with an infrared beam attached to a headpiece, performing grade level work academically.

Thoracic spine, ribcage, and upper extremities

Children with athetosis almost always completely bypass any weight bearing into the surface with their upper extremities. This may be for several reasons. The strong cervical and lumbar extension may lift such children in prone, or push them into the surface in supine, which substitutes for pushing with the arms. In addition, the arms often are placed in extremes of shoulder extension and internal rotation where the joint is most biomechanically stable. Because athetosis causes unpredictable generation of forces at unpredictable times, the child does not learn to rely on the arms for supporting antigravity postures. Also, the shoulder complex may assist head control with this strong elevation and shoulder internal rotation. This pattern to assist head control has been seen before in children with hypotonia and hypertonia, but tends to be even more pronounced in children with athetosis.

As the child is placed in the sitting and standing position or assumes them himself, the already flexed thoracic spine becomes a counterbalance for the forceful extension of the cervical and lumbar spine. In fact, the more the child tries to move using cervical and lumbar extension, the more he must compensate by flexing the thoracic spine so that he does not fall over. The child simply pulls harder into an already existing thoracic flexion posture, using strong shoulder internal rotation with the elevated shoulder complex. The pectorals and latissimus dorsi muscles become extremely tight.

Because the child with athetosis can and does move throughout extremes of some ranges when needed, she can assume a position of elbow extension with this strong shoulder elevation and internal rotation. What this child cannot do from this position is flex the elbow or supinate the forearm easily. The elbow is extended and the forearm pronated. She cannot rely on her neuromuscular system to give her consistent muscle activity, but she may be able to rely on the integrity of her musculoskeletal system to do so.

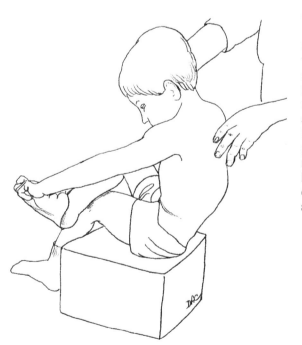

Figure 5.13 This boy with athetosis is trying to take his sock off. His thoracic spine is very flexed and his shoulder elevated with strong internal rotation. His elbow is in end range extension, which gives his arm some stability and consistent posturing. This use of joint integrity may be partially a learned use of the arm to make movement more consistent, because the child cannot rely on consistent muscle activity. His forearm is pronated.

With the above upper extremity posture, the only possibility for weight bearing on the hand is on the dorsum. Remember that the joints are not in midposition, as they are in children with hypertonia, but are instead at end range. If you hold your shoulder in strong elevation and internal rotation, full elbow extension, and full forearm pronation, your only choice is to bear weight on the dorsum of the hand.

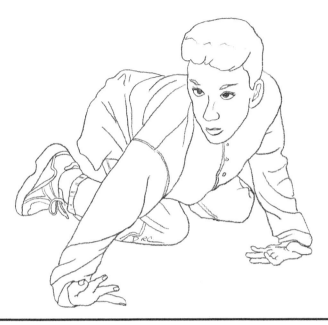

Figure 5.14 This teenager assumes an all-fours position with weight bearing on the dorsum of each hand. Note the eleva- tion of his shoulder complex and shoulder joint internal rotation.

The arm is moved from this position with shoulder abduction and internal rotation as the only possibility, and the movement is initiated with a change in position of the head. In fact, the head is used to initiate changes in limb position throughout the body and is an extremely important movement to look for and to understand in children with athetosis. Because these children often are unable to predict, antici-pate, or control the force and timing of muscle activity in the limbs, they develop a system to make posture and movement more predictable. This system is often one of use of the head, eyes, or jaw to increase the amount of flexion or extension bias in the limbs. Traditionally, these movements were called primitive reflexes and were seen as the release of lower central nervous system centers over movement control in children with cerebral palsy. They included the asymmetrical tonic neck reflex (ATNR) and the symmetrical tonic neck reflex (STNR). What many researchers and clinicians now feel is that these movements are not just stimulus-response patterns of movement or simply lower centers of the CNS controlling movement, but are perhaps the voluntary use of more easily coordinated patterns of movement to help solve a functional problem (Mandich, Simons, Ritchie, Schmidt, & Mullett, 1994; Pimentel, 1996). Therapists have more to learn about this, but in the meantime what the clinician sees is that children with athetosis learn to better predict the con-trol of the limbs by initiating movement from the head. It has been written that chil-dren with athetosis have the annoying habit of looking away from what they are trying to reach, as if this movement were one that the child uses to purposely avoid visual contact with people and objects or to make the learning of reach and grasp more difficult! The child actually is making reach easier and more predictable by turning his head, eyes, or jaw to initiate the arm movement. The severe price he pays for this is the inability to see what he is reaching for and therefore difficulty in accurately grasping and using what is in his hand.

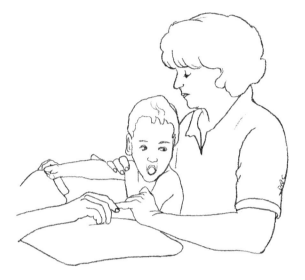

Figure 5.15 This boy uses head and eye turning with jaw extension to the left to reach for a toy with his right hand.

Mobility for arm movements comes from the movement of the scapula on the ribcage. The scapula can be mobile even though it is very elevated and abducted around the flexed thoracic spine, although it does not move into adduction or out of the elevation. The scapula has two reasons why it is not stable on the ribcage—it is poorly aligned, and it never had the development of thoracic extension with upper-extremity weight bearing to acquire stability.

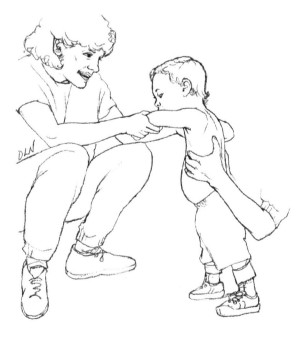

Figure 5.16 This child shows elevation, abduction, and upward rotation of his scapula with shoulder elevation and internal rotation.

Any ability to reach and grasp uses wrist flexion to a certain degree, often with metacarpophalangeal (MP) joint hyperextension. Various dynamic or structural changes occur in the interphalangeal (IP) joints, either in extremes of flexion or extension. The most common position seen at the proximal IP joints is hyperextension with a subluxed joint and slipped extensor hood. The intrinsic muscles of the hand are not used to control hand position or palmar arches do not develop. The child may use head and trunk flexion or extension to help flex or extend the fingers.

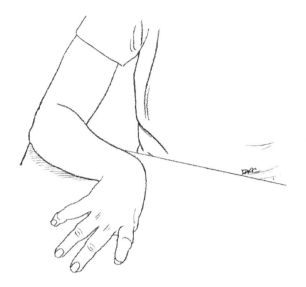

Figure 5.17a This teenager is attempting to reach for and grasp the front edge of her wheelchair tray. Her wrist is flexed and ulnarly deviated. All finger joints in the index finger are flexed, while the middle two fingers are extended at all joints. The fifth finger is not in extremes of ranges in its joints.

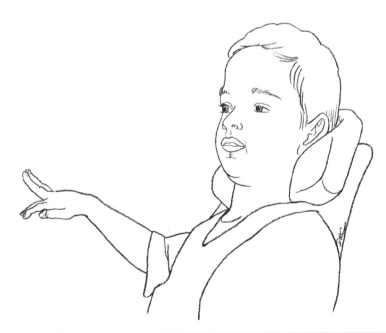

Figure 5.17b This child with athetosis is reaching for a switch to activate a computer. His wrist is flexed with his shoulder slightly internally rotated and his forearm pronated. In order to lift his fingers to place them on the switch, he extends at the metacarpalphalangeal joints of his ulnar fingers using the long finger extensors. Eventually, this overuse to the end range could result in subluxation of the joints.

One can imagine that the ribcage is very rigid. Remember that in children developing without disability the ribcage expands and changes shape as the thoracic spine extends, controlled lateral movements with rotation of the thoracic spine begin, and the abdominal muscles anchor the ribcage distally as the ribcage descends from its elevated position. In the child with athetosis, the thoracic spine has increased flexion, the entire spine moves in large, uncontrolled patterns of flexion and extension only, and the abdominal muscles are overlengthened with the elevated ribcage and the strong lumbar extension. The intercostals remain very tight, as does the structure of the ribcage. The ribcage may become very flattened anterior-posteriorly because many children with athetosis spend a great deal of time in their original hypotonic period lying on their backs or stomachs with little ability to move. In addition to the impairments of arrythmical breathing and poor timing of respiration with swallowing and voicing, the child cannot shift to thoracic expansion for breathing and does not have the mobility to rotate the thoracic spine, let alone control the rotation.

It is possible for the child with athetosis to learn some movement skills, despite the postures and movements described above. Movement in prone is almost always impossible or is severely limited. Given the above information about the upper body, one can see how hard this would be. Some children may be able to kick and push with their feet enough to scoot on their stomachs a short distance, but this is time consuming and energy costly. The thoracic spine is so rounded and the arms usually flail about, so that this area of the body interferes rather than helps. A more efficient way to move on the floor is by scooting in supine. Here the child does not need the arms to help the movement—she can kick and push with the legs while the cervical and lumbar spine extend. She can even see where she is going by extending her head with asymmetry. Besides, for the child with athetosis, it usually is easier to breathe in supine than in prone. The movement in supine is backward—the child pushes with the legs and moves back. Imagine what this may do to visual perception—the child learns about the world visually upside down and backward.

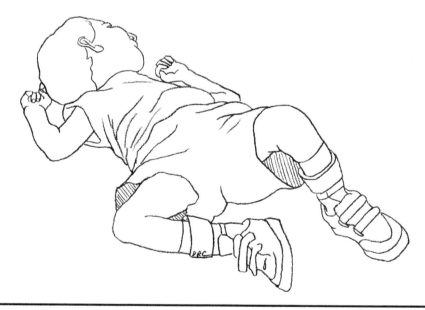

Figure 5.18   When scooting backward in supine, this 5-year-old looks up over his head with asymmetrically positioned eyes. If this posture and movement is repeated frequently and persists for months to years, what secondary impairments in visual perception develop?

Chapter Five

Another possibility for the child with athetosis in movement looks impossible to anyone else. It is the ability to move from prone to W-sitting. The child lies prone with the hips widely abducted. He uses a strong pull of flexion with the head and thoracic spine into the floor, thereby shifting weight to the upper body. He can flex the hips so that the legs are very close to the center of mass. After this, the child quickly and forcefully extends the cervical spine and lumbar spine to sit up. This enables the child to learn to sit up without ever having to rely on any upper extremity pushing. The mobility of the hips and the forceful flexion and extension of the spine enable the child to do what most other people could never do.

It is with grasp and manipulation that the child with athetosis will usually be the most disabled. Either her arms must lock into the position described in this section and move only with shoulder elevation, abduction, and internal rotation, or she must allow the unpredictable alternations between flexion and extension from the same shoulder complex posture to attempt reach and grasp. The first option may make the arm itself more stable and predictable in its movement, but does not enable anything more than pushing against something with the back of the hand. The second option may enable a gross reach, grasp, and release, but the arm trajectory can be unpredictable and very time consuming as the arm moves sometimes toward the target and sometimes away from it, even though the intended attempt is always toward it.

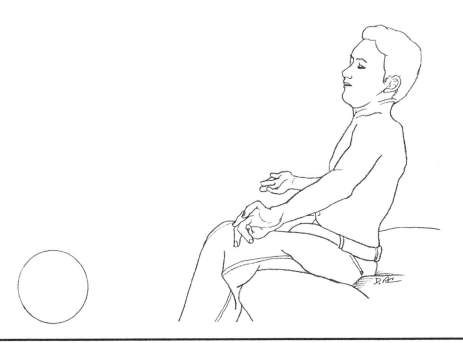

Figure 5.19 This teenager pushes a basketball from his lap. His shoulder complex elevation, shoulder internal rotation, elbow extension, and forearm pronation enable him to contact the ball with the dorsum of his hand only. He moves the shoulder with abduction—the only possible movement he can make from his starting position (try it yourself).

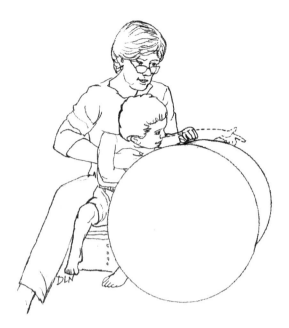

Figure 5.20 This child attempts to reach for a toy that his mother is holding on the opposite side of the therapy peanut. The trajectory of his reach is unpredictable and alternates between a flexion and extension movement at the elbow and hand.

Functionally, the child is limited severely in arm use for postural support, movement transitions, and reach, grasp, and manipulation. Also, the thoracic spine must work very hard in flexion to counterbalance the strong cervical and lumbar extension, so cannot do anything else. The child cannot expand the thoracic ribcage for respiration.

Children with athetosis have many severe disabilities as a result of these functional limitations. An 8-month-old cannot prone prop, belly crawl, creep on all fours, sit with upper extremities free for play, or make sounds as she plays. She also can only reach with a swiping motion, often making no contact with a desired toy and never able to grasp or manipulate it. A 2-year-old can reach with his right hand only when well supported in an adaptive chair. He can grasp the toy with the radial side of his hand in contact with the tray of the chair, and tries to manipulate with the ulnar fingers.

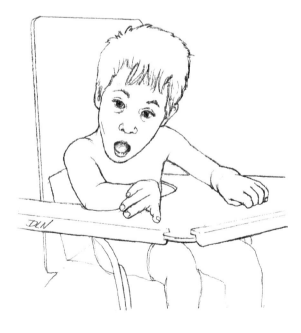

Figure 5.21 With shoulder internal rotation and forearm pronation to the end of the range, the radial side of this child's hand is the weight bearing or supported portion. He then learns to try to grasp toys with the ulnar side of his hand.

He can only do a gross grasp and release this way and gets very frustrated that he cannot make the toys do what he wants them to do. He cannot do any type of self-feeding, including finger feeding. He can scoot about the floor on his back, but this is his only form of mobility. He makes a breathy "ahhh" sound to call attention to himself and to indicate a yes response, but has no other way to indicate desires or needs. A 5-year-old can bunny hop, propelling herself with a lifting of her legs while her arms are non-weight bearing. She can W-sit, yet is unable to use her hands to play with toys.

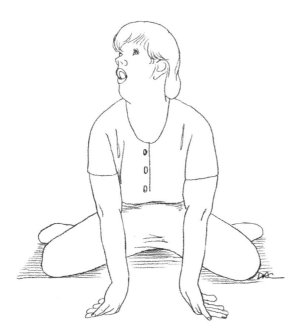

Figure 5.22 This older child W-sits with a very wide base of support using hip abduction with internal rotation and her feet dorsiflexed. She rests her hands on the floor so that they will not flail about, but does not take any weight on them. To *bunny-hop* forward she lifts her lower body with her hip adductors and medial hamstrings, then thrusts her lumbar spine into extension as she scoots her legs slightly forward.

She can push keys on a computer keyboard with a key guard while in her wheel-chair, and is doing kindergarten-level games on the computer. She cannot voluntarily phonate and often cries when she wants something and no one can figure out what it is.

An 8-year-old who is learning to drive her power chair understands how to work the joystick and probably could learn how to steer because she understands the concepts of movement of her body through space and direction changes. But each time she places her hand on the stick and tries to push it, she has to turn her head away from the arm that is pushing, and so cannot see where she is going. She has learned definite movement patterns since she was a baby—her head and arms move as a unit. To lift and move an arm, she always turns her head slightly away from the arm.

Children With Athetosis

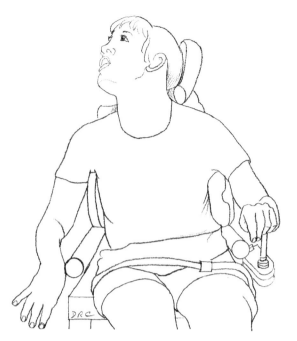

Figure 5.23 This child turns her head away from the arm she reaches with. This asymmetrical cervical extension is the only way she knows how to initiate reach. As she begins to try to drive her power chair with this movement, she is unable to see where she is going.

A 13-year-old can do standing transfers with the assistance of people familiar to him, but cannot help in managing clothing in the bathroom. He indicates needs on an alphabet board that he points to with the index finger of his right hand. His wrist flexes and the MP and IP joints hyperextend. He can say about 10 words that people who are familiar with him can understand. He cannot feed himself and is learning to use an infrared head pointer on a communication system.

In children with hypertonia, remember that with the effort of trying a difficult skill, the children often become more stiff, and therefore, even more unable to perform. In children with athetosis, the effort and desire to perform is not only very frustrating to them, but often increases the extraneous movements that interfere with skill acquisition. (Remember that in Hallett and Alvarez's study, increased effort often increased activity in the antagonist.) Because children with athetosis often are keenly aware of the skill they are trying to perform or that others want them to try, this can become an incredible obstacle to success. I have seen several teenagers who desperately wanted to learn at least some self-feeding. They worked hard with their families and occupational therapists to find the best way to do so. They learned to scoop up pretend food with a spoon or fork, bring it to their mouths, and managed to get it in the mouth. But when it came to trying the real thing, the excitement and knowledge that it was real made them unable to achieve success.

Lower trunk

The child with athetosis often develops lumbar extension simultaneously with cervical extension. Because the thoracic spine is rounded and rigid, the extension often occurs almost exclusively at the thoracolumbar junction. (This biomechanical advantage to thoracolumbar extension is described thoroughly in the section on children with diplegia on pages 122 and 123.) The child often works the lumbar extensors very hard. Remember that the child is lifting or pushing with the upper body with this extension without any assist from pushing with the arms. If the head is lifted with marked asymmetry to one side, the child also may show asymmetry in the lumbar spine, setting up the likelihood of developing scoliosis and hip dislocation.

In supine, the child often looks as if he is bridging the hips because the extension is so strong, but the extension is strongest in the lumbar area, not the hip joints. Again, if the child is asymmetrical, the functional scoliosis that results will influence hip position as well as that of the trunk (see Figure 5.4 on page 148).

Given such strong use of the lumbar extensors and the elevated position of the ribcage, the abdominal muscles are poorly aligned to be used posturally because they are overlengthened. Therefore, there is no stability of the base of the ribcage anteriorly.

The superficial extensors of the lumbar spine can become very shortened. This includes the erector spinae, the quadratus lumborum, and the latissimus dorsi.

While children with hypotonia and hypertonia may extend the lumbar spine in some postures and flex it in others, the child with athetosis who uses strong extension to attempt antigravity movements often uses extension in the lumbar spine in all postures. The exceptions are children who are still very floppy with only some athetoid movements seen distally in the mouth and hands. They may be unable to generate the antigravity extension in the trunk to try to move, and therefore, flex throughout the spine in all postures. These are usually children with the most severe impairments and disabilities.

Functional limitations result when the lower trunk has only one choice for movement and postural control. In the child with athetosis, the strong lumbar extension with no stability from the abdominal muscles severely limits how the child can control the center of mass. The lower trunk does not have the option of controlling weight shifting with cocontraction of flexors and extensors to hold the center of mass stable. Nor can the lower trunk flex with extension of the thoracic spine as the center of mass moves toward the back of the base of support in a posterior weight shift. The lower trunk cannot cocontract to assist the entire trunk in lateral movements, either. The lack of synergy selection also limits respiratory control—the abdominal muscles cannot perform the functions of holding in abdominal contents and resisting the diaphragm during inspiration and cannot grade activity to control expiratory rate.

Disabilities result from having only this one option to control the lower trunk. A 5-month-old not only cannot prone prop because of lack of arm use, but cannot breathe well in prone because the abdominal muscles cannot help lift the ribcage and abdomen off the surface as the child also lifts the head. Therefore all of the child's weight is taken on the belly, which he needs to expand to breathe. (Many children with any type of cerebral palsy have this problem to a certain extent, and therefore do not like the prone position.)

A 4-year-old not only sits with a rounded thoracic spine in a supportive chair, but sits more on one hip than the other as his lumbar spine asymmetrically extends. He develops redness of his skin on the hip and thigh that he sits on, and is becoming more intolerant of sitting.

A 16-year-old is hospitalized frequently with pneumonia, missing his schoolwork and other daily routines. One reason for his frequent pneumonias seems to be his poor respiratory pattern and his poor ability to generate a forceful cough.

The pelvic girdle and lower extremities

Remember that the child with athetosis starts life as an extremely floppy baby. If placed without any support in all postures, the child's head tends to fall completely to one side, completely forward, or completely backward. The arms and legs are in a frogged posture. It's not just a frogged posture as seen some premature infants—this abduction of the limbs with flexion approximates 180°. The upper extremities may be limited somewhat in this abduction because the shoulder complex is so elevated at birth that the arms can't spread out. This is seen in any position the infant is placed (see Figure 5.9 on page 153).

As the child begins to move antigravity with strong cervical and lumbar extension, the legs provide a wide, stable base of support for this movement. While the arms tend to fly around or are held with strong shoulder elevation and internal rotation away from the surface, the legs can anchor the trunk as it moves in prone and supine. Children with athetosis tend to spend prolonged time in these positions, since they do not develop control of more antigravity postures. The child can count on the position of his legs, which is always the same, to assist attempts at antigravity control. It usually is true that children with athetosis are better with their legs than their arms. The legs are in a predictable position and actually provide some positional stability to initial postures, whereas the arms are unpredictable and unreliable in their postures and movements. The consistent, weight-bearing position of the lower extremities decreases extraneous, non-functional movements. It is not uncommon for children with athetosis to have almost no arm function, but they can stand with one person assisting them and take steps if someone supports their trunk. They also may learn to move in their wheelchairs or on the floor using the more predictable movements of their legs to propel them. This was illustrated in the movie *My Left Foot* (Conroy, 1990). The young man first showed his family that he could write by using his foot. Although he was described as spastic and may have had some spasticity, his primary postures and movement patterns, impairments, and disabilities were those of a person with athetosis.

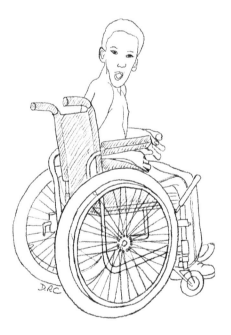

Figure 5.24 This 13-year-old cannot use his arms to propel a manual wheelchair. However, he has used strong asymmetrical head turning and pushing with his feet to propel himself in supine on the floor in the past. He simply adapts this pattern to propelling the chair—he turns his head to see behind him, then pushes on the floor with his feet. He can only move backward, although he may become proficient at maneuvering and turning this way.

What the child learns to do from the initial starting position of hip flexion, abduction, and external rotation is use bursts of flexor and extensor activity in the legs to push the feet against the floor or other support surface. The child usually does not get into the hip flexion, adduction, and internal rotation seen in children with hypertonicity, at least at first, because of the initial position of such wide hip abduction. The knees remain in some degree of flexion during this pushing and the feet often are dorsiflexed and everted.

The initial position of the hips also may help keep the child from developing scoliosis, at least for a while, because the base of support for lifting the trunk is so wide and symmetrical. However, if the child starts lifting and pushing in supine or when seated, the asymmetry that starts from the head will eventually affect the trunk position and ultimately the hip position. For example, the child may learn to scoot backward in supine using symmetrical movements of the lower extremities to push and propel with. As she looks to see where she is going, using even more cervical extension asymmetrically, the side of the trunk on the face side is elongated and the side of the trunk on the skull side is shortened. This causes the pelvis to lie asymmetrically, with the shortened side elevated and the lengthened lifted from the surface. The hip follows, becoming less abducted and externally rotated. As the child lifts and pushes this way, she stretches the anterior portion of the hip capsule and ligaments.

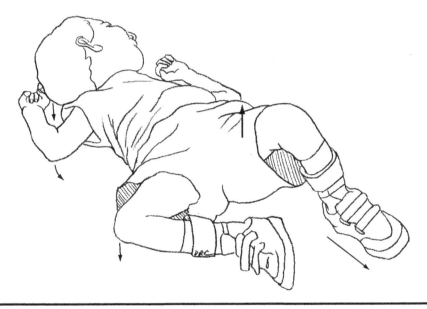

Figure 5.25 This 5-year-old with severe hypotonia and athetosis is pushing himself back in supine. As he lifts his hips up from the surface using extension in his cervical and lumbar spine from an asymmetrical starting position, he places stretch on the anterior hip joint. If he repeats this movement over years, especially if his extension becomes stronger and more asymmetrical, he could eventually anteriorly dislocate one or both hips.

The child with athetosis can push hard this way. Although the anterior capsule and ligaments of the hip are very strong, years of pushing can weaken this area. The hip can dislocate anteriorly as a result. Because of the mechanism described to dislocate the hip anteriorly, it is usually a problem only seen in older children or adults with athetosis.

As the child with athetosis learns to assume and move in other postures besides prone and supine, the hip and the rest of the lower extremity postures can vary. For example, the method for getting into a W-sitting position has already been described. When the child assumes W-sitting, the hips switch from a position of external rotation to one of internal rotation by virtue of the movement of the trunk and pelvis over the hip joints.

Because the child with athetosis has more mobility in the hips than the child with hypertonia, the total posture in W-sitting looks different in the two children.

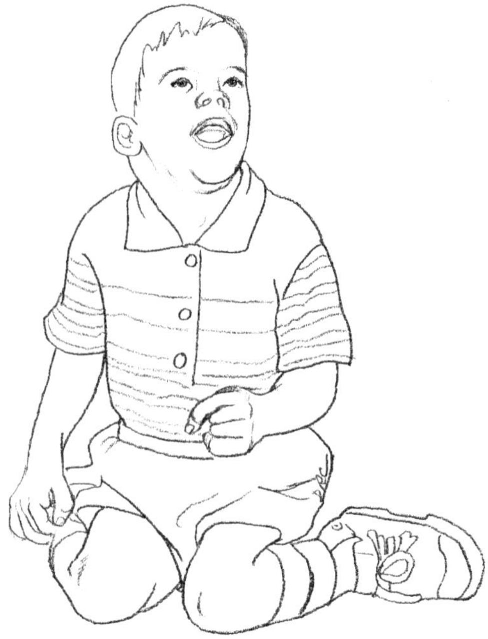

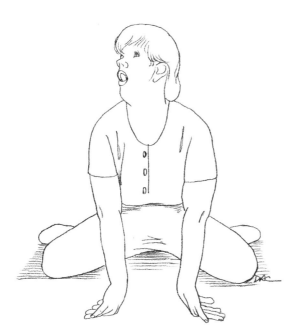

Figure 5.26 This child with spastic diplegia W-sits with hips in internal rotation and adduction.

Figure 5.27 This child with athetosis W-sits with hip abduction and internal rotation. Her base of support is wider than the child who has diplegia and her lumbar spine is more extended, whereas the child with diplegia postures the lumbar spine in flexion.

The child with athetosis may learn to bunny hop from this W-sitting position. He uses the more reliable, wider-based legs to initiate and control movement. He uses the adductors with internal rotation from an abducted position to first lift the body. Then there is some sort of wiggling or scooting using flexion/extension movements from the lower extremities, trunk, and head to move forward. The arms do not participate. The most they may do is rest lightly against the floor so that they do not fly around during forward movement.

The child also may learn to pull to stand. If the child can bunny hop, she can move to a stable piece of furniture and rise up into a sort of kneeling position by lifting the body with the lower extremities. She can place one arm on the furniture, initiating this movement with head turning, then place the other arm on the surface by turning the head the other way. Once the arms are on the surface, the child puts the forehead or chin against the surface (certainly this child is not going to rely on her arms to pull her up). By pressing down with the forehead against the surface of the furniture and pushing with the lower extremities into extension with assist from the hip adductors, the child may be able to get into the standing position.

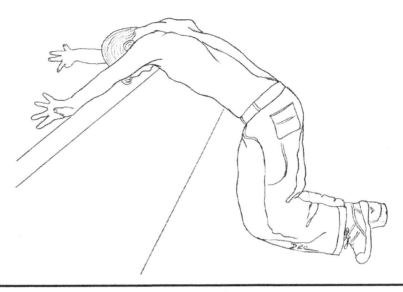

Figure 5.28a This 13-year-old with athetosis is able to pull himself to standing using heavy furniture for assistance. He lifts himself from the position in Figure 5.14 into a kneeling position using contraction of his hip adductors and extensors. He then places his forehead on the edge of the couch and presses it down (the way other people would push with their arms). This helps support his body weight and enables him to first move his legs a little closer to the couch, then to push his feet against the floor.

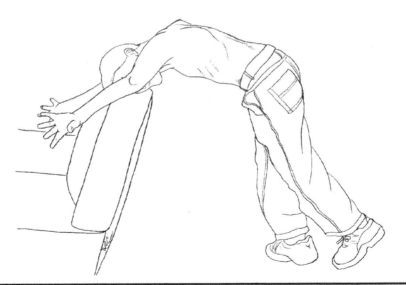

Figure 5.28b The boy can now use extension in his legs to stand plantigrade and can step closer to the couch. He still takes considerable weight on his forehead and/or cheek. Little to no weight is taken through his arms. Now he faces a difficult task—how to stand up completely. He needs to move the long lever arm of his entire upper body over his lower body.

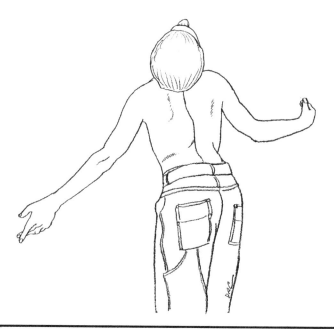

Figure 5.28c To accomplish the task of moving the upper body over the lower body, he relies on strong cervical and upper lumbar extension with no power from his arms. No wonder many children with athetosis cannot stand up by themselves—this movement requires strength and control of trunk extensors to lift the long lever arm of the upper body over the lower body.

Some children with athetosis can learn to stand and walk independently. (Although this chapter has focused on children who are severely physically affected, because that is the most commonly seen, some children are more mildly affected. They may learn to walk, talk, and use their arms to a certain extent. Their biggest disabilities tend to be in the areas of hand usage and speech intelligibility.) Their posture is classic. The thoracic spine is very rounded with the arms often clasped or crossed in front of them to prevent losing balance backward. The arms also are clasped to control their unwanted movements. The hips and knees are flexed slightly, and the feet are dorsiflexed. They often shuffle their feet to progress forward, using head, eye, or jaw movements to initiate weight shifting. If they were to shift weight the *typical* way, completely unloading one leg to swing through, the supporting limb would collapse. This is because of the unpredictability in the force production and timing of the muscles supporting the one leg. So instead, the child with athetosis keeps both feet on the floor at all times and keeps the base of support wide, and uses small degrees of head, eye, and/or jaw movements to shift weight just enough that a foot can move forward slightly.

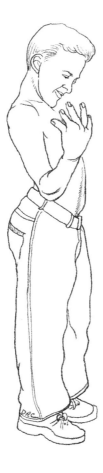

Figure 5.29 This 13-year-old with athetosis stands with strong end range lumbar extension and a thoracic kyphosis. He sustains his head in an active chin tuck to further ensure that his lumbar extension does not knock him over backward. His hand appears very large in this drawing because his elbow is held tightly at his side, his shoulder is slightly externally rotated, and his wrist is flexed (the hand is coming straight at the camera in the photo from which this picture is taken).

More mildly affected children can walk faster and more efficiently by flexing their hips instead of their thoracic spine. This compensation prevents the overpowering cervical and lumbar extension that are likely to knock the child over backward.

Functional limitations that result from the lower extremity movement compensations in children with athetosis include a lack of reciprocity of movement due to the inability of the trunk to actively rotate, combined with the initial wide base of support from hip positioning, as well as the primary neuromuscular impairments. The legs are used for stability, not for controlled mobility. If the stability function were removed without work to improve trunk function, the child would not be able to assume and maintain most of the postures she can control. Therefore, as the therapists treat the child, lower extremity position and base of support have the possibility of change only when functional trunk activity increases.

Disabilities can be illustrated as follows: A 13-month-old can stand supported by his mother, although he sometimes collapses, especially if he drops his head forward into flexion. Yet he cannot assume or maintain sitting independently, crawl or creep on the floor, or roll.

A 3-year-old can sit when placed in a wide-based ring-sitting position, but falls over backward if she holds her head erect (she must keep it dropped forward to stay sitting). She cannot assume or get out of any sitting position herself. She can scoot backward in supine, pushing with her feet. She can stand at a walker with a tray to place her arms on, as long as she can keep her elbows extended and grip around the edge of the tray. If she lifts a foot to try to step, she usually collapses.

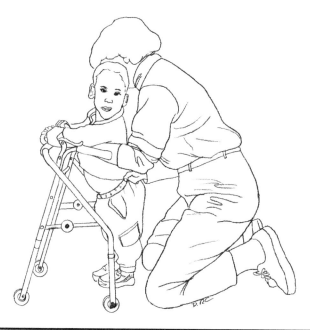

Figure 5.30 This child is able to stand with assistance at a walker if the arms are supported in elbow extension with shoulder internal rotation. This position then requires the child to grip the front edge of the walker frame or the tray supporting the arms.

A 9-year-old can transfer in and out of his wheelchair with someone supporting his trunk. He can take steps with this support, but has never been able to use any type of assistive device to walk.

A 15-year-old can bunny hop on the floor and pull to stand at his wheelchair, but cannot turn around to seat himself in the wheelchair independently.

General Treatment Strategies

Children with athetosis start out very floppy as infants with an asymmetrically positioned head and wide-based extremities. They learn to move against gravity as their motor control allows by using strong bursts of extension that often quickly die out. The movements are not only asymmetrical, but also forceful, and usually through wide ranges. As a result, the child has a very abnormal sense of midline.

This child also learns early to have a little more control of flexion and extension distribution and force throughout the body by changing the position of his head. Head and arm movements are strongly connected—often inseparable. He may control lower body flexion and extension, as well as hand and jaw opening and closing, by changing the position of his head. This further impairs visual skill development.

The therapist—whether physical, occupational, or speech—must be concerned first with the child's inability to separate head, eye, jaw, and arm movements from each other. This affects virtually any functional skill. Treatment must begin with centering the head and eyes while building more postural control in the trunk. Because young children with athetosis often are able to follow simple verbal instructions and want to use their eyes to learn with, motivation usually is not a problem. Therapists often start in a position in which they do not have to control the whole body, but rather have their hands free to help position and hold the child's head, support the arms

Chapter Five

in weight bearing, or place toys. I like the prone position on a very large ball because I can bring the child to an almost upright position, which is better for development of head control than a horizontal prone position, but enables upper-extremity weight bearing.

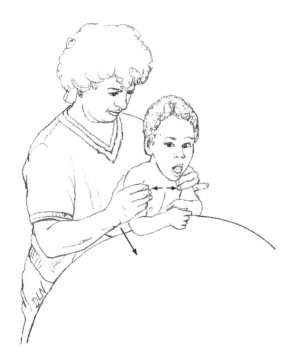

Figure 5.31 This child's therapist sandwiches him in between her body and the ball to fully support him. She then aligns his shoulders in more flexion and external rotation while firmly pushing down into the ball. Now she will encourage him to first visually fix straight ahead on something of interest to him, then to begin visually following in small ranges. His mother might be holding a book or favorite toy in front of him.

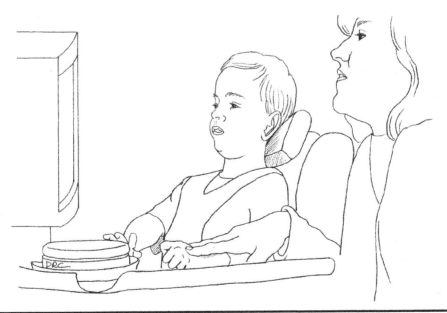

Figure 5.32 During this child's therapy session, his therapists are helping him visually fix on the computer screen while push-ing a switch. His wheelchair is used to support head and trunk alignment so that the therapist can assist more distal function.

Children With Athetosis

After positioning the child in midline with the above trunk support, ask him to begin turning his head while his arms remain in weight bearing (with help initially). The head and the eyes move together at first, and later the eyes slightly lead the head movement. The child will probably open his jaw as he first tries this, losing ideal head alignment.

There are times that you can support the arms in weight bearing and also help control head position.

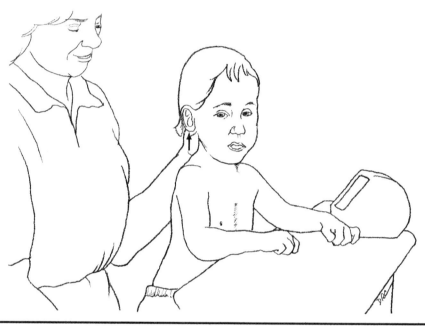

Figure 5.33 This child with athetosis is finally able to rest his arms quietly on the bench in front of him, although he does not yet take weight through his arms on his own. His therapist now helps him grade head turning to search for a toy. She sits behind him and supports his lower body position with her legs, then gives traction to his cervical spine to help him bring his head in flexion on an extended cervical spine. She uses the web space of her hand firmly on his occiput to do this. From this position, she can help him grade cervical rotation as he visually searches.

After you play games that enable the child to more freely move the head while keeping the body relatively still (often with adaptive equipment assist and support), begin to help him move his arms while his head stays relatively still. You want him to focus on a toy or person while supporting the head as necessary, and reach for something that you feel he can be successful with. Do not expect accurate reach at first or a totally quiet body, especially the jaw. The child must first learn that he can initiate arm movements without so much overall body movement and certainly without turning the head completely away. This teaches him that he can still see what he is reaching for. Although this may seem out of the realm of possibility for many children with athetosis, many children can learn to do this. They can at least learn to turn the head and eyes through a smaller range of movement while they reach so that they can maintain visual contact with what they are reaching for.

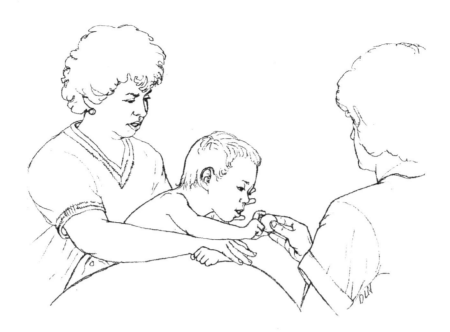

Figure 5.34   This child is helped to reach for a toy as he maintains eye contact with it. His therapist has first helped him achieve weight bearing on his arms and a more midline position. She continues to support one arm in weight bearing and also limits the movement of his head with her other hand as he reaches.

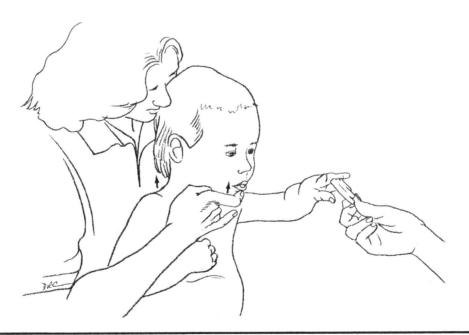

Figure 5.35   This child with athetosis reaches for a cookie. When doing this unassisted, he turns his head to the right and opens his jaw with forceful extension. His therapist supports his head with one hand on his occiput and the other gently supports his mouth closed with oral control. She gives him this control before he even sees the cookie, since he anticipates the reach with his asymmetrical extension posturing.

Children With Athetosis

Begin to work for the function itself—reach and grasp with visual guidance, grading jaw opening and closure on a cracker, standing transfers with upper extremities supported on therapist's shoulders, and so forth. It is absolutely necessary to start with the separation of head, eye, and arm movements for almost any skill that the child and the family want the child to learn.

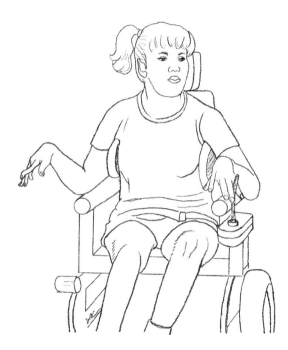

Figure 5.36 This 17-year-old with spastic athetosis drives her power wheelchair. She is able to look at the hand that controls the joystick and can look in front of her to see where she is going.

Pay attention to the child's learning a way to quiet his forceful, non-functional movements. Many children with athetosis can learn on a cognitive level to quiet themselves when preparing for difficult movements or skills. Since this quieting is on a cognitive level, however, I find that the child cannot do it all of the time—no one can think continuously about their posture and movements and expect to function in the real world. However, the child can learn a signal, such as "it's time to get quiet" prior to performing a skill that is especially difficult. It often succeeds in preparing the child's posture initially so that initiation of the movement or sustaining of a posture is possible for skill execution. With practice, this quieting becomes a part of their motor learning, and is therefore a more automatic part of their posture and movement without so much verbal instruction.

Choose your words carefully as the child and you work together to help her learn a new skill. The child with athetosis often knows what is expected of her and has ideas of how to do it. Therefore, choose instructions that she may not anticipate. Anticipation often elicits a non-functional burst of movement that you want the child to avoid. Be one step ahead of this anticipation initially to avoid the huge emotional and physical burst of activity that she would try on her own if not guided. For example, do not say to a child with athetosis, "Stand up now." If you say that, especially if the child is not optimally aligned with the hips flexed well past 90 degrees, the result is that she attempts to stand with a huge burst of extension, pushing backward and taking the therapist with her. Instead, help the child flex the hips well past 90 degrees, place her arms on your shoulders, lean her forward over her feet, and say something like, "Come toward me and then up." The difference is not only in the preparation of the body, and in dividing the skill into specific movement components, but in the words used. To a child with athetosis, the word "stand" means to use all the extension you can. Instead, choose words that mean the same thing, but do not elicit the emotional and physical response.

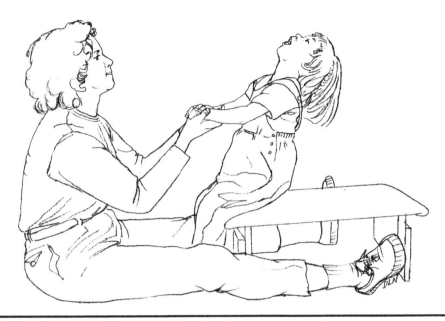

Figure 5.37 This child with spastic athetosis is asked to stand up. Her response is to use strong cervical and lumbar extension with lower extremity extension while her center of mass is well behind her feet. The result is that she moves up and back.

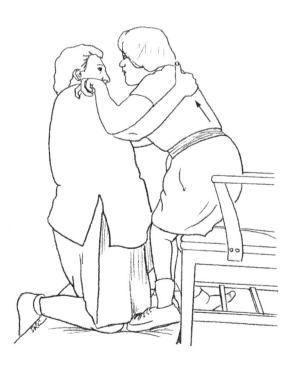

Figure 5.38 When asking this teenager to stand, her therapist first prepares her alignment with as much thoracic extension and hip flexion as possible. If possible, try to flex the hips past 90° prior to standing (it is not possible for this girl). Only after her alignment is prepared is a verbal request given. You may want to say "Come toward me and then up" instead of "Stand."

Another example may be helping the child to eat. If the child sees the food that he is about to eat, then shown that it is coming toward his mouth, it is already too late to think that the therapist is going to help him learn to grade jaw opening and closing. The child's jaw is already fully opened at this point with extension of the legs so that he is practically standing in his chair. Instead, this is a time when you may not want the child to anticipate what is coming. Position the child well, placing your hands in a way to assist oral control, then present the food at the moment you want the child to take a bite. You are likely to be positioned behind and to the side of the child. Once the food is there, then you can say "bite," or use some other verbal cue. Eventually, of course, the child has to be presented with the real situation of eating, but at first you must eliminate the emotional and physical cues that cause him to be out of control before you even start.

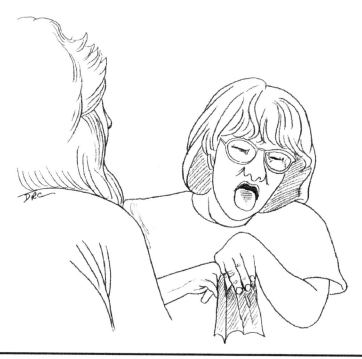

Figure 5.39 As this teenager sees food presented to her, she extends her jaw and protrudes her tongue. She is already in a position now that is very difficult to correct to allow graded oral movements.

Chapter Five

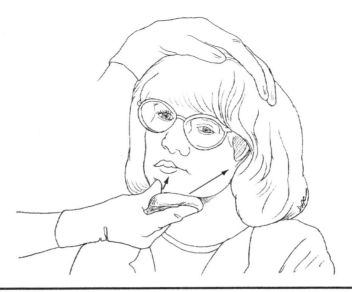

Figure 5.40 The teen's therapist spends a few minutes prior to feeding her to prepare her oral area as seen here. She gives prioprioceptive information through her temporal mandibular joints followed by graded release of her jaw to allow the teen to take over controlled jaw opening and closing. The therapist then approaches her from the side, offering food while simultaneously saying "bite" so that the girl becomes more automatic with her biting rather than spending a prolonged time anticipating taking a bite.

In working with children with athetosis, I usually can help them align their trunks more functionally and have better balance of flexion/extension activity in the trunk. This means that I must often spend time helping the pectoral and latissimus muscles elongate in order to help the thoracic spine move into more extension.

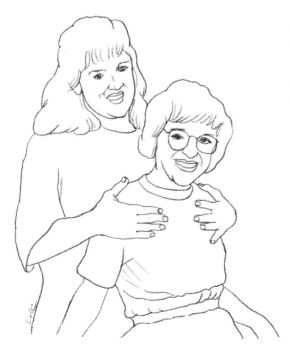

Figure 5.41 This girl is working on sustaining thoracic extension while her therapist lengthens the pectorals. The therapist opens the width of the upper chest as the hands are slowly moved along the muscle in parallel with the muscle fibers. The therapist may abduct her own fingers for additional stretch. Once she reaches the shoulders, she can move her hands laterally around the arm just below the shoulder joints as she externally rotates the shoulders. Shoulder external rotation facilitates thoracic extension.

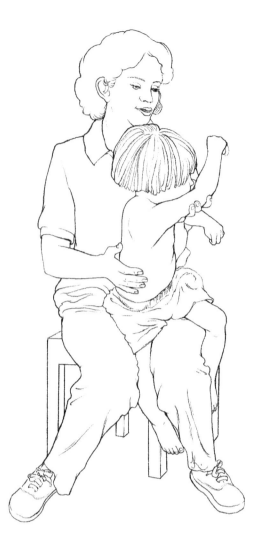

Figure 5.42 This child is working actively with visual fixation on a toy, active assistive thoracic extension with rotation, and assistance to help her terminate sustained latissimus dorsi muscle activity and/or lengthen the latissimus muscle. The therapist applies downward force at her ribcage with her right hand while assisting thoracic extension and rotation. She gives gentle sustained traction to the child's right arm with her left hand to put the latissimus muscle in its lengthened position.

With the trunk erect and the shoulder girdle more optimally aligned, it is possible to help the child into a position of some degree of thoracic rotation. Ask for active work while holding this rotated posture—it helps prevent the child from forcefully extending the body backward and enables him to possibly use more balanced flexion and extension activity to control the trunk. This works especially well when sitting and flexing the hips past 90 degrees.

A good example of this is a child, often with spastic athetosis, who can talk but who cannot use the arms for anything functional, actively assist in movement transitions, and so forth. The way he initiates and sustains breath support for talking, which he does all day, ruins the possibility of learning any other skills. This is a child who initiates voicing using eye, jaw, cervical, lumbar, and lower extremity extension, then sustains breath holding to force out the words. He can say only two or three words per breath, and must repeat the process. This effort to speak limits the number of words he can say in a given period, so his speech pathologist may want him to be able to say more words, and intelligibly, per breath. His PT and OT may want to know how to help him control respiration as he talks while he moves. You want his body in a position that eliminates the possibility for this massive extension to force out air. You may choose to put him in sitting with the hips flexed greater than 90 degrees, his thoracic spine extended and rotated, prior to asking for voicing. Help support the abdominal muscles for assist with breath control. Finally, ask him to initiate voicing as he looks at you rather than up at the ceiling.

Chapter Five

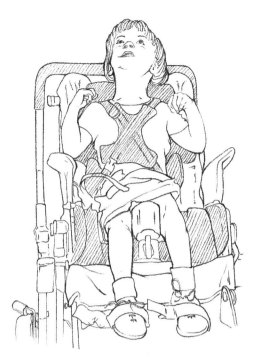

Figure 5.43 This child with spastic athetosis initiates voicing by pushing out her exhalation with lumbar, cervical, and eye extension. As she does this, her limbs stiffen with cocontraction.

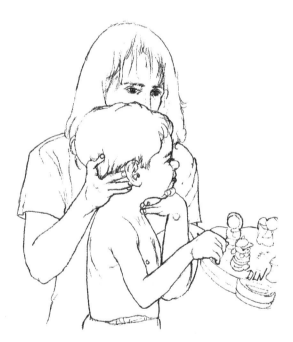

Figure 5.44 This child's speech pathologist gives him oral control and support to his head as she asks him to voice. She has him positioned in at least 90° of hip flexion with thoracic extension prior to this facilitation. As he voices, she encourages him to look straight ahead at his mother, who is on the other side of the toy.

In working with the lower body, you want the legs to be aligned so that movement transitions and weight shifting in sustained postures can be accomplished with more ease. You and the child have to work together to find a way to first just keep the legs quiet and in place. The use of joint approximation, weighting the legs in good alignment, and practice shifting the upper body over a stable lower body that you help keep in place are often good techniques. I usually find that strapping the legs in place in adaptive equipment only results in the child's body fighting against the restraints. On occasion, however, some children have allowed me to lay sandbag weights across their thighs when they are seated.

To conclude, let's look at two children with athetosis and follow a treatment sequence that a therapist might use to accomplish a functional skill. The first is a 5-year-old who wants to learn to feed herself by bringing food to her mouth with a fork. The therapist wants the child to bring the food to her mouth after the food has been stabbed onto the fork for her, put the fork into her mouth and take off the food, then chew and swallow it. The child has the most difficulty with the part of the skill that requires her to bring the food to her mouth and get the fork in her mouth. Each time she quiets the arm enough to allow the process to begin, she has to turn her head away from the arm holding the adaptive fork (a fork that doesn't require an active grasp) to flex the elbow. Then as the food nears her head, she drops her head down toward the fork (if she stays erect as she brings the food to her mouth, her experience is that her cervical and lumbar extension cause her to lose her balance backward). By the time the fork is near her mouth, her chin is practically on her chest and she cannot get the fork in her mouth.

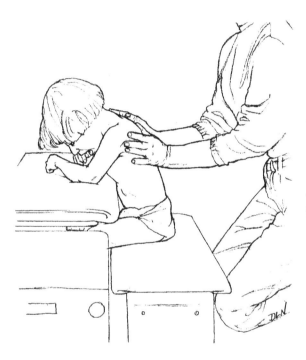

Figure 5.45 As this child brings her hand to her mouth to feed herself finger foods, she drops her head down. She does this because she has experienced that bringing her hand up toward her mouth causes her to fall over backward (her cervical and lumbar extension is unbalanced in her trunk). This compensation of bringing her head forward results in poor orientation of her mouth to a hand that cannot release in this position.

The child in this common situation must be able to visually guide the arm throughout the feeding process and keep the head and trunk erect enough that her mouth is in a position that can at least be capable of receiving the fork. You may play some games first with the child without the use of the fork and food to help establish postures and movements without the stimulus of the food. First work to achieve thoracic extension and decrease shoulder complex elevation, if necessary, while keeping the hips well flexed in a sitting posture and feet quiet on the floor.

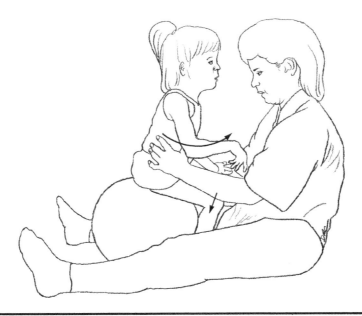

Figure 5.46

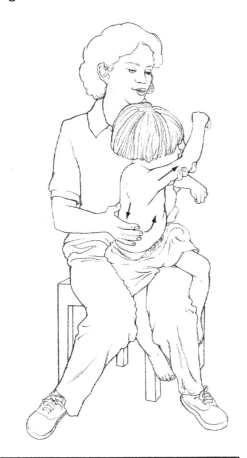

Assist reaching from a thoracic extension/rotation position for a ball (about 8–12 inches in diameter) or other toy to play a game. Assist reach and grasp as needed. Play a game where the child can keep the elbows relatively extended, since this will probably be easier, but demand visual attention with a fun game. Assist trunk and head posture and support the reaching and grasping arms as necessary. Make the game harder each time.

Now she must bring the ball up against her chest before throwing it. Assist elbow flexion with shoulder complex out of elevation and without losing the trunk and head posture.

Figure 5.47

Then she has to touch her nose with the ball before throwing it. After this, switch activities so that she is given the fork with no food yet. Ask her to touch her mouth with the fork, but that is all. Verbally and physically reinforce the erect trunk and head with visual guidance

while helping her isolate elbow flexion for the fork to mouth movement. She will do best if she places her elbow in weight bearing on a table or tray to learn this movement. Finally, she may attempt to bring the fork, now with food on it, to her mouth.

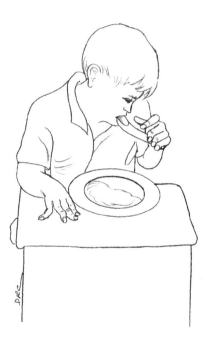

Figure 5.48   This child is very much like the child in our case study. He also is 5 years old and has athetosis. After intense work by his occupational therapist, using treatment progressions similar to the child in our case study, he began to be successful getting the spoon to his mouth. He sits with a fairly erect trunk and can lightly place his right hand on the table. He still turns his head and lowers it a bit to reach the spoon, but he also is able to lift the spoon part of the way to his mouth and can look at what he is doing. He therefore is successful part of the time in obtaining food such as yogurt, applesauce, and mashed potatoes from the spoon. His OT will continue to assist him in isolating head and trunk posture from upper extremity movement for the goal of faster self-feeding, less messy feeding, and to feed himself more difficult foods to scoop and retain on the spoon.

Select her home program based on how easy it is for her to accomplish hand-to-mouth movement. If she still has a great deal of difficulty and you must help facilitate much of the posture and movement control, ask her family to play the ball game with her at varying degrees of difficulty while she sits in her wheelchair. Show the family how to help her bend her elbows and hold her hands against the ball. Remind them that the game involves hands to head rather than head moving toward hands. They may be able to find a fun, competitive way for siblings to play to keep the game interesting.

If you find a way to simply hold her shoulder, elbow, or wrist to help her eat while she is well seated, then show the family this as a home program.

The second child is a 9-year-old with athetosis who can walk independently. He wants to learn to dribble a basketball in his physical education class and at home with his brothers. Every time he stands and holds the ball, he grips it tightly as he tries to stand still. He flexes his neck to help him hold onto the ball and to prevent loss of balance backward in standing. When he tries to let go, which takes a lot of time, he has to turn his head with extension and rotation to release the ball. When he does this, he loses sight of the ball. The result is that he can bounce the ball once, but cannot hit it again as it bounces back. The ball usually goes in one direction and his eyes and body are off in another.

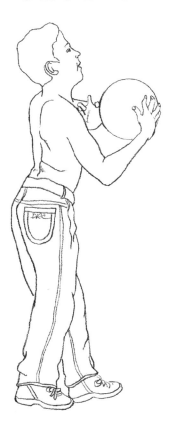

Figure 5.49 The child begins to release the ball. He is unable to release the ball as he looks up with his head in midline.

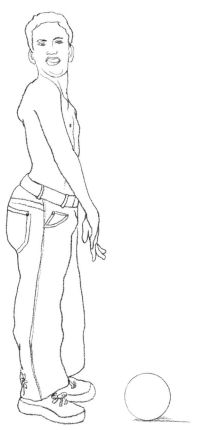

Figure 5.50 To release the ball, he has to extend his cervical spine and then turn his head. When he does this, he cannot maintain eye contact with the ball.

This child needs to learn to grip less forcefully and to let go of the ball without so much head turning if he is to have a chance at beginning to dribble the ball. To facilitate the learning of better head and arm coordination, you may have him begin by sitting on a bench, to counteract the problem of controlling his body while standing. While seated, you can assist trunk posture with alignment and joint approximation through the trunk, then ask him to hold the ball as he looks at it. He then has to just drop the ball at a target—not throw or bounce it.

Then he may work to throw the ball with the target a short distance away so that he can't be successful if he is too forceful. Encourage visual attention.

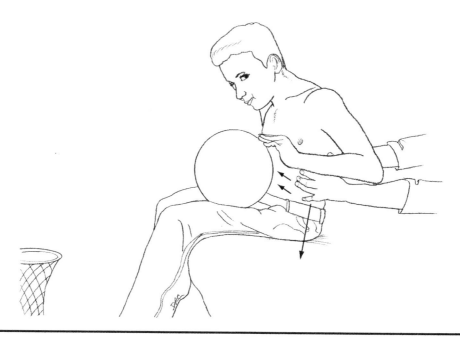

Figure 5.51   As his therapist supports his lower trunk and uses joint approximation to help him actively hold, she asks him to place or throw the ball into a hoop located in front of him on the floor. He is sitting on his bed. Sitting takes away the difficulty of controlling the standing position and the drop or throw decreases the force he needs when releasing the ball.

Then he may stand and do the same skills. You can assist standing stability with lower body alignment and joint approximation.

C A S E   S T U D Y   *(continued)*

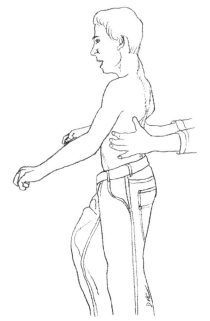

Figure 5.52   Now, the same progression is assisted and repeated while standing.

Ask him to drop the ball and catch it when it bounces up while he looks at the ball. He has to turn his head and eyes a little, but recovers quickly enough to catch the ball as it bounces back. Work to increase the speed. Now he is on his way to learning the skill, as the main obstacles of his posture and movement problems have been decreased.

Ask the boy's father to practice these new bouncing and catching skills at home, suggesting that they mark off a square in the grass or on the sidewalk as a visual assist to guide where the ball goes and where the boy needs to look.

CHAPTER SIX

Children With Ataxia

Pathophysiology

Children with ataxia (from the Greek *a* + *taxis*: no order) probably have damage to the cerebellum or possibly to any of the pathways that provide cerebellar input or output (Bastian, 1997). Ataxia also can result from peripheral lesions that damage the ability to sense or perceive proprioceptive information. In cerebral palsy, however, we are concerned with cerebellar ataxia, not the types caused by peripheral lesions.

In children with cerebral palsy, the incidence of ataxia is reported at less than 10% (Esscher, Flodmark, Hagberg, & Hagberg, 1996). These researchers report that within this population of children with non-progressive ataxia, there is probably a high proportion of children with familial, genetic causes of their ataxia. There also may be children who appear to have a non-progressive ataxia and are diagnosed as having CP but who turn out to have a progressive or genetic disorder that remains undiagnosed despite extensive testing from well-qualified physicians. In the study done by Esscher et al. (1996), 61% of the 78 identified children with ataxia did not show any abnormality at all on their neuro-imaging tests.

Several clinicians have questioned whether ataxia should be considered a type of cerebral palsy. Although the term *cerebral palsy* in no way describes the type or severity of the impairments and disabilities that children experience, the problems in children with ataxia are very different from those with other classifications of CP and many of these children may have other causes of their ataxia than CP. The problems in ataxia are so different that there are many clinicians who have little experience in identifying and treating children with it. If we better identify these children, we may find that the incidence of ataxia is much higher than 10%, or at least it may be one of the classifications of CP in a larger number of children with mixed types of cerebral palsy than we currently identify.

Let's look at some of the terminology used in the literature to describe children with ataxia.

> **Ataxia:** Failure of muscular coordination; irregularity of muscular action (Dorland's, 1994). An inability to coordinate muscle activity during voluntary movement, so that smooth movements occur. Most often due to disorders of the cerebellum or the posterior columns of the spinal cord; may involve the limbs, head, or trunk (Stedman's, 1995).

> **Dysmetria:** A condition in which there is improper measuring of distance in muscular acts; disturbance of the power to control range of movement in muscular action (Dorland's, 1994). An aspect of ataxia, in which the ability to control the distance, power, and speed of an act is impaired. Usually used to describe abnormalities of movement caused by cerebellar disorders (Stedman's, 1995).

Tremor: Repetitive, often regular, oscillatory movements caused by alternate, or synchronous, but irregular contraction of opposing muscle groups; usually involuntary (Stedman's, 1995).

In general, ataxia means a lack of coordination with tremor and dysmetria present. But all children with CP have difficulties with coordination, so the term *ataxia* does not help with understanding the differences between children with ataxia and other children with cerebral palsy. In addition, not all children with ataxia tremor, especially very young children. Some older children may tremor very little or only under certain conditions. And although dysmetria is fairly well defined, clinically it can be hard to tell whether the child doesn't smoothly reach a target because of this disorder of power, speed, and distance caused by a cerebellar lesion, or whether she has trouble with power, speed, and distance because of other multiple impairments.

To sort out the problems in the child with ataxia, look first at what the cerebellum is presumed to be responsible for. This provides information on the negative symptoms that may be possible in children with ataxia (the impairments). The cerebellum seems to be responsible for many important functions. It times and organizes motor commands, especially rapid movements. It monitors and updates evolving movement. It predicts movement in feedforward and preprogrammed movements with occasional proprioceptive input. It is responsible for helping coordinate smooth visual pursuits. It interprets and routes proprioceptive and vestibular information. It subtly adjusts complex patterns of coordination by comparing what actually happened to the original plan (the basis of motor learning). It also may be responsible for the timing and ordering of some cognitive processes (Doyon, 1997; Hallett and Grafman, 1997).

Children with ataxia often show delayed initiation of movement, loss of terminal accuracy (dysmetria), saccadic dysmetria, intention tremor, poor adjustments to sensory discrepancies or to proprioceptive information, and exaggerated responses to some sensory information. These children are extremely disorganized (lack of motor learning capabilities and poor timing of muscle contractions are possible causes). They also are extremely fearful of movement, especially movement that involves subtle action in the trunk. This is even so for those who seem to bounce off the walls all day. They rely heavily on trying to establish visual stability—if they have not done this, they usually do not move much at all.

In summary, children with ataxia, in general, are very disorganized in their movements and cannot rely on proprioceptive and vestibular information to help them learn about their world. Because of the poor timing of muscle activity, they cannot rely on consistent muscle responses. So they make one of two choices—either not to move much at all or to blunder headlong through space. Their skills may vary from one day to the next. Some days they can sit in a chair and some days they fall off the chair repeatedly. Teachers report that these are children who know the alphabet one day and do not seem to know it the next.

The consistent thing about children with ataxia is that they seem to be inconsistent. Skills or movement components that appear similar to us vary so much in context for this child. But when the child's sensory and motor learning impairments and functional limitations are more thoroughly understood, the inconsistency makes sense. For example, the child can stand if supported by his mother, but cannot stand while holding onto furniture. An onlooker might observe that the child is just being lazy or manipulative because he stands so well by his mother, and the furniture offers just as much support. However, if evaluated carefully, the clinician notes that the child is fearful of new situations, and standing by furniture is new, whereas standing by his mother is something he has done for many months. When standing by his mother, she holds him firmly and close to her, perhaps giving him the necessary visual and proprioceptive information he needs to feel confident of standing.

Standing by furniture gives the child little proprioceptive information about body position in space and visually may look as if he is standing suspended in space.

Children with ataxia, like all people, must learn skills in the context they will need to use them. Yet the child with ataxia has a great deal of difficulty generalizing any part of one skill to another skill. Other children with cerebral palsy can learn movement patterns, and some of the general qualities of those movements easily carry over into similar functions. For example, a child with diplegia can learn how to step up onto a folded mat with his crutches to learn the skill of stepping onto a curb rather than go outside on a rainy day to learn on a real curb. Then the next time he goes outside to practice, he usually readily remembers how to place the crutches, how to shift his weight, and so forth. In a child with athetosis who gets so emotionally excited or so goal-oriented that she cannot perform well, simulating a function works well to teach the function itself. For example, the child's occupational therapist may use hard plastic bracelets to teach a child how to put on the sleeve of a jacket. The hard plastic is an easier material to work with than a soft jacket, but involves a very similar pattern of movement. This strategy often carries over well when the therapist tries the real thing after the child masters the basic pattern of movement with supporting postural stability.

These two approaches seldom, if ever, work for a child with ataxia. If you want the child to learn to put on a coat, he must have his actual coat to learn the skill. If you are teaching him how to negotiate steps, then you must go to the steps he will be using. All foods are new foods to a child with ataxia, and any food may be rejected because the child sees no consistency between foods with some similar and some different characteristics (taste, color, texture, temperature). For therapists in hospitals and clinics, this makes the treatment for this type of child much more of a challenge than for those treating in schools and homes.

Again, in this chapter we will describe children with pure ataxia. There probably are many children with mixed types of cerebral palsy who have some component of ataxia. Hopefully, this chapter will give insight into the unique and profoundly disabling impairments seen in children with ataxia so that these features of the movement disorder can be identified in children who have mixed types of CP.

Impairments

Neuromuscular system

Reflexive tone

Reflexive tone may present as normal or slightly depressed deep tendon reflexes (DTRs). In many problems associated with lesions in the cerebellum, hypotonia is frequently mentioned (Rosenbaum, 1991). If depressed DTRs accompany this hypotonia, then it may make sense that in children with ataxia, one finding could be depressed DTRs.

Difficulties with muscle contraction

Children with ataxia show delayed initiation of movement. Movement initiation could be delayed because agonist activity is reduced in force (Bastian, 1997). Sustained movement may be very difficult for the child with ataxia because of the lack of continuous, low-level muscle fiber firing normally regulated by the cerebellum. These children certainly have difficulty terminating muscle activity. There is evidence that people with ataxia may prolong antagonist activity, so that there is delay in termination of movement as well as delays in the initiation of the agonist (Bastian, 1997). There also is the common observation that children with ataxia show hypermetria—the overshooting at the end point of movement, which may be considered a problem with timing and grading movement (Rosenbaum, 1991).

Grading agonist/antagonist activity

In children with ataxia, there often seems to be an ability to use patterns of cocontraction and reciprocal inhibition, but the timing and smooth gradation are abnormal. In Nashner, Shumway-Cook, and Marin, (1983), the classic study of postural responses on a platform with various alterations in sensory conditions, children with ataxia showed normal abilities in use of cocontraction and reciprocal inhibition in postural responses. Responses were consistent across trials.

Hallett, Shahani, and Young (1975) showed that in patients with cerebellar disorders, a task that required rapid movements at the elbow between flexion and extension resulted in abnormal timing of the triphasic burst of agonist-antagonist activity. In people without disability, a rapid movement is performed by a characteristic agonist-antagonist-agonist triphasic pattern of activity. In the patients with cerebellar dysfunction, none of whom had congenital ataxia, however, the triphasic burst, although present, showed a prolonged initial burst of the agonist or a prolonged burst of the initial agonist, then prolonged antagonist activity. This correlates with hypermetria (overshooting) (Hallett, et al., 1975). If this is typically true of children with congenital ataxia, then what we may conclude is that consistent and normally sequenced agonist-antagonist activities exist, but the timing of these contractions, and probably the intensity of them, are abnormal.

Many children with ataxia learn to use cocontraction voluntarily to prevent movement of their center of mass. Their neuromuscular systems seem to give them this option, and they use it to prevent movement that they know they cannot control. They also increase the use of cocontraction with fear of movement and use cocontraction if needed to lower the center of mass toward the ground. It is because children with ataxia can do this that they are sometimes initially diagnosed with spastic diplegia. However, if observed carefully, children with ataxia, when they feel secure, use a much wider variety of movement patterns than children with diplegia. The child with ataxia resists passive movement voluntarily, not because of its velocity. It may take some time to see these differences, however. Of course there are children with both diplegia and ataxia, so this complicates things even more!

Limited synergies used to produce posture and movement

Perhaps children with ataxia lack the ability to use some muscles or muscle synergies with correct force because they do not regulate muscle activity or correct force production when multiple joints need to work together (interaction torques) (Bastian, 1997). Clinically, it appears that many children with ataxia use the right muscles to try to perform postures and movements, but they do not time the contractions well. Nashner et al. (1983), found that children with ataxia used the correct synergies of movement in postural sway in stance perturbations, but that the latencies for muscle contractions were prolonged and variable.

Certainly in the clinic, children with ataxia look different than children with other types of cerebral palsy, often showing normal-looking muscle mass and body segment proportions. In other words, it is difficult to see the disability, because physically these children resemble children developing normally. This may be because children with ataxia use their muscles in a variety of synergies and frequently enough that muscle bulk and limb size develop fairly well. This is both a blessing and a handicap—it is great to have the children we treat develop the musculoskeletal system well, but when society at large cannot see a physical disability, they often tend to believe there is none present.

Sensory/Perceptual systems

Children with ataxia often have profound problems using visual information to learn about their world. And yet, this often seems to be the best sensory-perceptual system they have, so in treatment I use their vision to help teach them more about function. I also treat their visual system according to its needs.

Recall in Nashner et al. (1983) that children with ataxia used normal synergies of movement in the right order, but with prolonged latencies and variability in those latencies. Children with ataxia showed the motor component of their postural adjustments to be the closest to normal of any of the classifications of cerebral palsy. However, their performance was often the poorest in Nashner's study, with frequent falls and large amplitudes of postural sway. When visual conditions were altered so that the visual surround (walls of the room) moved while the floor did not, the children with ataxia swayed excessively or fell. Children under age 6 and adults with vestibular dysfunction respond similarly. Visually, the room is perceived as moving, even though through the integration of all sensory systems, the body orientation is not moving. The conclusion of the researchers was that children with ataxia have deficits in central sensory feedback mechanisms, which perceive motions of the body with respect to gravity and the surrounding environment. This is a primary impairment in the somatosensory system. They also hypothesized that the intention tremor seen in ataxia may be a result of this abnormal feedback system rather than a problem with coordination in the motor system.

What is clinically relevant from this study and from clinical observation of children with ataxia is that they believe their visual system—whether it gives them accurate information or not. Therefore, therapy must help them organize consistent, meaningful visual information so that their worlds become more stable and meaningful. Yet children with ataxia often have motor nystagmus (the rapid, oscillating movements of the eyes) that decreases visual acuity and causes them to alter head position to visually fixate. They also may come to therapy initially with extremely poor visual attention—they don't focus or maintain gaze on anything, shift gaze, or track objects. Smooth visual pursuits are one of the primary functions of the cerebellum, and it is therefore no wonder that children with ataxia have difficulties tracking. But the visual system of children with ataxia often is their best system in the learning of postural control and movement gradation, so I concentrate very hard on this system.

Children with ataxia may learn to use upward visual gaze or excessive visual fixation to try to stabilize their posture (the latter child is at least one step ahead of the child who cannot use visual fixation). They may hold their heads very rigid and move their eyes with their head exclusively rather than leading head movement with the eyes. All of these could be secondary impairments as the child tries to learn to stabilize the world visually. However, they also may be primary impairments because the cerebellum is responsible for minute corrections of head and eye movements when focusing on an object and for visual anticipation of movement. What happens clinically in many children with ataxia, is that they can respond and learn from first learning to fixate on objects, then learning to shift gaze while they are stationary, then learning to visually scan while their heads move but their bodies do not, and then learning to visually scan while they move. The last and hardest component that some children with ataxia are able to master is the ability to use downward gaze while they are moving (parents of such children frequently complain that not only do they never seem to look where they are going, but they are in extreme danger on the stairs, simply walking off the top step and falling down).

In treatment it is absolutely essential that you work on the visual components of movement with children with ataxia if they are going to learn new skills. Changes usually can be made here.

Children with ataxia seem to have a profound loss of the ability to use proprioceptive information. This clinical observation can be supported by the knowledge that the cerebellum is responsible for the interpretation and routing of proprioceptive information. In addition, in Nashner's et al. (1983) study the problems of children with ataxia were believed to be due to central processing problems of all sensory systems—the study did not attempt to sort out one system from another.

Children with ataxia often have a very poor ability to learn through the proprioceptive system. Try joint approximation techniques through well-aligned joints in these children because sometimes it does help, but not nearly as well as it helps children with other classifications of cerebral palsy. There often is the confusion expressed by therapists that they do not know whether they are treating a child with athetosis or ataxia—they see uncontrolled, excessive movements that may be tremors or choreoathetosis. I advise them to look elsewhere. Concentrate on how the child uses and learns from her sensory systems. Children with athetosis usually learn well through their tactile and proprioceptive systems, whereas children with ataxia do not. Children with athetosis can generalize motor learning to similar skills, whereas children with ataxia often cannot.

Children with ataxia often do many things that seem alarming to observers and are attributed to poor behavior or lack of parental control rather than to their sensory-perceptual problems. They bite hard on many objects, including people. They approach their toys with grabbing movements, then throw their toys after banging and mouthing them. They stuff food into their mouths and would choke if someone didn't monitor them. They store food between their gums and cheeks, sometimes for hours. They try to eat inedible objects, such as the paper that surrounds a candy bar. They rub their mouths on rough surfaces. All of these behaviors tell me that the child is having a tremendous problem perceiving proprioceptive and tactile information. Of course, hitting and biting are behaviors that we do not let others do to us and they must be addressed as inappropriate in children with ataxia as in any other child, but at least we can understand why this behavior often is used. The child with ataxia has to learn that he cannot hit others, though he will not understand that hitting hurts.

Children with ataxia are likely to have impairments that affect the vestibular system. We know that the vestibular system is closely linked to the cerebellum since the cerebellum processes and routes vestibular information. In addition, studies such as Nashner's et al. (1983) showed that children with ataxia behave like adults with known vestibular problems in their postural responses. The difficulty is trying to sort out which system in children with ataxia is responsible for the disorganization problems they have. This can be almost impossible. Take a very organized approach to treating children with ataxia that includes organizing visual and vestibular information to help give them postural stability. Using linear vestibular input can be organizing for children, so incorporate this in treatment during meaningful motor skills.

Children with ataxia often show profound auditory processing delays and impairments. It is not unusual to get a response to a question long after the question is asked. Although this is a clinical observation only, it makes sense that children with ataxia have this impairment because so many of the other sensory systems show problems in central processing.

Although there are estimates that children with ataxia show about a 60% incidence of mental retardation (Esscher et al., 1996), I wonder if it is really possible to accurately test such children. Because of their profound and multiple sensory processing problems, formal testing must be extremely difficult. Recently, Schmahmann (1991) reviewed 264 research reports concerning altered intellectual and behavioral functions in animals and humans with cerebellar lesions. He discusses the anatomical connections between the cerebral cortex and the cerebellum and describes studies done experimentally with animals and clinically with humans with known cerebellar lesions. He cautiously states that we need to pursue more work in this area to determine the possible connection between cerebellar lesions and deficits in higher intellectual processes. Doyon (1997) and Hallett and Grafman (1997) also review recent research with the cautious conclusions that the cerebellum most likely has some role in cognitive processing.

Musculoskeletal system

Children with ataxia tend to have the least difficulties in the development of this system in comparison to children with other classifications of cerebral palsy. This may be because they use a variety of movement synergies to perform functional skills, and so secondary impairments are less likely to develop. Children with ataxia who are more hypotonic tend to show some of the musculoskeletal impairments that children with hypotonia do. This is especially seen in an elevated and rigid ribcage and some tightness of the superficial muscles of the trunk. There may be pronated feet with weight bearing and quite mobile joints in the hands.

Sometimes some of the limb muscles become shortened. This is because many children with ataxia can make themselves quite stiff. They stiffen the joints through the use of cocontraction to try to decrease the movement of the center of mass. They also may use excessive cocontraction to lower and hold the center of mass closer to the ground, again to prevent movement that they fear they cannot control. This, then, can result in some muscle groups becoming tight from constant use and positioning. It is not unusual for children with ataxia to be mistaken for children with diplegia because of some of the posturing they do with their legs. However, the posturing is much more under voluntary control and is seen when they are fearful and not when they are more comfortable with their postural support and stability.

Children with ataxia may show some minor congenital deformities. This has been reported in the literature (Miller, 1989) and leads researchers to question the complexity of ataxic CP. Again, the possibility exists that very early neurological and embryological events are important determinants of the outcome of children with cerebral palsy. The congenital anomalies that Miller found include high arched palates, minor malformation in the hands and feet, epicanthic folds of the eyes, and minor structural malformations in the ears and nose.

Children with ataxia usually do not have major impairments in the development of strength. Again because of their abilities to use a variety of movement synergies and the ability to use patterns of cocontraction as needed, most muscles can develop the strength necessary for functional tasks. The more the child spends time not moving at all, or holding himself rigidly in midline to prevent movement of the center of mass, however, the more likely it is that some muscles will not develop normal strength throughout full range. The most likely muscles to show weakness are the postural muscles of the trunk needed for controlled weight shifting and rotation and support of respiration.

Respiratory system

Children with ataxia have difficulty timing respiration with voicing. Their respiration is usually shallow with belly breathing the predominant pattern. There is lack of emphasis on syllables of words, making the speech monotone. There is a marked delay in the onset of voicing with each attempt to speak. Words are spoken slowly. Speech is often dysarthric, perhaps because of the poor sensory awareness within the mouth, the shallow respiratory pattern with little use of abdominal activity and intercostals to help grade exhalation, and the delayed initiation of muscle activation.

Many children with ataxia do not produce more than a few vocalizations. Although it can be difficult to evaluate just how much cognitive deficit is part of this observation, it is clear that motorically many children with ataxia have enough impairments within the oral area and in respiration to make sound production limited. It is not unusual to see a child with ataxia who can only make a few vowel sounds and perhaps a "ba" sound. Yet that same child may be able to communicate on a higher level with sign language or other forms of alternate communication.

Secondary impairments that result from the sensory impairments and lack of postural muscle activation include a rigid ribcage, often with a flattened anterior- posterior diameter, distal ribcage flaring and structural changes to the ribcage over time, a mild thoracic kyphosis, usually with elevated shoulder complex, and often a forward head posture.

Typical Posture and Movement Strategies
Head, neck, tongue, and eyes

The child with ataxia usually starts as an infant who has a tendency to be slightly hypotonic (some children who go on to show signs of ataxia later are quite hypotonic as infants). Because of this early development on a hypotonic postural base, many children with ataxia develop their postures and movement control patterns very similarly to children with hypotonia.

Like children with athetosis and some children with hypertonia, the positive signs of ataxia do not usually appear until well after the first year. These signs include tremor and dysmetria with poor accuracy of termination of movements. However, I may begin to suspect that an infant will show these signs later and will become ataxic if I observe several characteristic behaviors that are different than those of children with pure hypotonia. These are the severe sensory-perceptual problems. So, in addition to noting if a child learns to hold up her head by placing the occiput back on the spine, uses musculoskeletal stability to hold up the head, has an elevated shoulder complex, a passively retracted tongue, and eyes gazing upward, I am likely to begin noticing issues of a more sensory-perceptual nature.

When the child is fed, he has a tendency to choke excessively. Food may be stored in the mouth without the child's awareness that it is there. He will begin to mouth objects, but unlike children developing normally, he will mouth toys and other objects in his environment excessively and exclusively—not only does everything go in the mouth, but that's all he does with it. He drools profusely and seems not to notice. He may rub his mouth on rough surfaces and bite hard on anything he can put into his mouth. When he begins feeding himself, he will tend to overstuff his mouth, chew poorly, and have difficulty using active lip activity to clean a utensil or the oral area. These observations do not always mean that this child is later going to be ataxic, but they are red flags.

Some children with ataxia use the same postures described for children with hypotonia but tend to avoid any oral contact with toys or food. They seem tactilely defensive both inside and outside the mouth. They are usually children who do not vocalize much. Again, these are not problems that are exclusive to children with ataxia but are problems to note for the present and compare to future development. At this point, in addition to a detailed description of how the child interacts and the postures and movements he uses, there are signs of poor sensory awareness and poor development of perceptual skills.

Children begin to show clearly that they are ataxic when they do not use their sensory systems to learn about movement and to monitor posture and movement control.

When they do not look at what they are doing, they approach objects or people with excessive force. However, if they do look at something they approach and are familiar with, they may grade force quite well (another example of their seeming inconsistency). Their play strategies are very limited, despite motor skills that would enable more variety to their play. They show their ataxia in the slow, monotone speech or in the inability to coordinate respiration with voicing well enough to produce more than a few sounds. They may begin to show tremors of the head and eyes (nystagmus), but these are not always present or obvious.

Probably the most obvious movement problems involve the use of the eyes and head to monitor postural stability and movement control. Children with ataxia show several distinct ways of moving when they have a severe problem with processing sensory information. One way is just not to look at anything for very long, with eye movements that seem fleeting, uncoordinated, and unable to hold a gaze. These are usually children who have some ability to move about a room, but constantly trip, stumble, fall, and run into everything. They are described as hyperactive and are mistakenly thought of as children who love to move. They never look where they are going. As a therapist, your biggest challenge is to catch the child first, then try something that will slow him down! That something is visual stability.

Another common finding is a child who seems much more cautious. This child has found that to move, she must find a place to visually fixate, usually somewhere across the room, then stare at that point as she makes her way through the room. This may be similar to the way all of us walk across the deck of a boat that is pitching on the waves—we pick a point on the stable horizon and go for it. The problem is that we see nothing in our path. This is exactly what happens to this child—she sees nothing in her path because she is not visually scanning, just staring. So she bumps into, trips over, steps on anything in the way. This gets such children into trouble not only physically, but often behaviorally as they step on their preschool classmates as they make their way across the room.

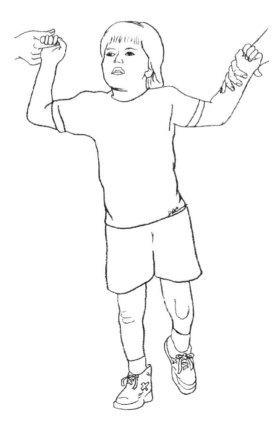

Figure 6.1 This 8-year-old with ataxia walks with his hands held. He cannot walk independently. He uses upward visual gaze and stares across the room as he is led through his classroom.

The other option is a child who doesn't move much at all. This child can often sit when placed and maybe even creep on all fours, but cannot walk. The child may use fleeting eye movements that seem to disrupt his fragile postural control as he sits or he may visually fixate on something and just not move. If he does move, he moves very slowly. This is a child who would stay in one place for hours if someone else did not move him. When someone does try to move him, he is terribly frightened unless he is familiar with either the person or the assisted movement.

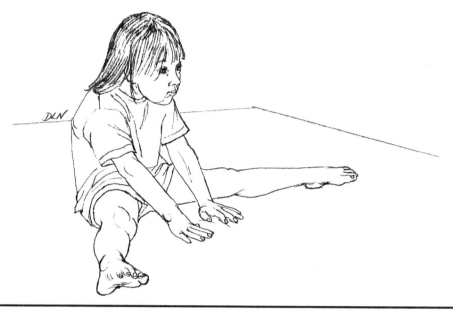

Figure 6.2   This child sits with thoracic flexion and a wide base of support. She is hypotonic and ataxic. She is able to visually fixate on something, which she uses to assist her in sustaining her posture. Without visual fixation, she tends to tremor more and can even fall from this sitting posture.

The other clear distinguishing characteristic of children with ataxia is their excessive drooling, mouthing of toys and other inappropriate objects, and biting and tearing of toys with their teeth. Certainly drooling and mouthing are not exclusive features of ataxia, but children with ataxia seem to bite and mouth exclusively with hard movement that lacks grading, even though they are physically capable of grading movements in other situations. Of course, to add to the complexity of this, there are children with ataxia at the other extreme—children who don't want anything near their mouths. But some of the other visual problems and sensory-perceptual problems throughout the rest of the body will help distinguish them as children with ataxia.

Functional limitations result from the reliance on musculoskeletal integrity instead of neuromuscular control and from the severe sensory-perceptual impairments.

Disabilities are illustrated in the next three children. A 10-month-old can sit when placed with cervical spine extended on an extended head, mild kyphosis of the thoracic spine, and legs in a wide base of support. But she cannot move in and out of sitting, pull to stand, or walk around furniture. She uses her hands as part of her base of support while sitting, and so seldom manipulates toys while sitting on the floor. Besides, she can't see them anyway, since her eyes are in an upward gaze. She eats well when fed, with occasional choking on liquids, but does not vocalize at all in any position. She seems to be passive, having no facial expression most of the time. She will occasionally turn her head slowly toward her mother when her mother calls her name.

A 3-year-old can walk and run. He climbs the stairs, but often falls. He tries to go down the stairs too, but his parents are terrified when they watch him—he looks straight ahead, then manages to go down a few steps haphazardly with poor coordination so that he looks as if he could fall at any time. He picks up toys and throws or bangs them on the floor, seldom looking at them. He eats independently, but overstuffs his mouth and chokes. His preschool teacher often finds some of his breakfast in his mouth 2 hours later. He has several words that people who know him understand, but his speech is severely delayed. He drools profusely and seems unaware or unconcerned about it.

A 10-year-old tremors both at rest and with movement, primarily in his head, eyes, and trunk. He is able to sit and creep on all fours independently and walks with a weighted walker; but he does not walk independently. He visually fixates on a target in order to reach as well as to move on all fours or in his wheelchair, all of which he does very slowly. He can do very little in the area of fine motor skills due to his tremor and poorly developed manual skills (sensory and motor impairments), but can use a computer with a keyguard on the keyboard. He speaks in phrases very slowly, but is generally understood by most people. When asked a question, he seems to take forever to answer, but when he does, he usually is correct. He is doing academic work on a second grade level.

Thoracic spine, ribcage, and upper extremities

As mentioned previously, children with ataxia often initially develop as children with hypotonia do. Therefore, it is typical to see infants and young children who will be ataxic show an elevated shoulder complex, mildly kyphotic thoracic spine, slightly extended and internally rotated shoulders, and an elevated, rigid ribcage. Because children with ataxia cannot trust the timing of their movements, despite the variety that often is available to them, they voluntarily hold their trunks very stiff and rigid to prevent as much movement of their centers of mass as possible. So while children who are hypotonic only may stay in a midline position with their trunks and sink into gravity, the child with ataxia who has more neuromuscular control of cocontraction and synergies will actively hold the trunk in midline.

This results in a trunk that shows an increase in the degree of shoulder complex elevation and ribcage rigidity over time as this child can hold it in position, whereas the child with hypotonia sinks into gravity. The trunks of children with ataxia can be unbelievably rigid. Most of the rigidity is active holding to prevent weight shifting, but there are secondary impairments that result. Range of motion loss into thoracic rotation and scapular depression often result. The pectorals and latissimus muscles shorten. The intercostal muscles are very tight, and the lumbar extensors may be tight. It is easy to see that this child, on first or superficial impression, is seen as a child with hypertonicity and diagnosed as spastic.

The child with ataxia usually has a variety of movements available for upper extremity function. The more elevated she maintains her shoulder complex, however, the more limited the possibilities become. Many children with ataxia can use the variety of synergies seen in children developing normally, with graded control and very little, if any, tremor. This can be very confusing when trying to understand why the child is so limited functionally. Other children with ataxia definitely show tremor in the upper extremities, especially with movement, and are limited in the movements themselves. In these children there is no question that they are ataxic. In addition to the tremor, they often overshoot their reach and have to work hard to correct arm position to place the hand where they want it.

What these two types of children with ataxia share are their profound problems using sensory information to guide and correct movements. So even though a child may use a variety of normal synergies of movement, especially when visually monitoring the arm, he has characteristics that show he is not sensing or processing somatosensory information well. This is a child who only bangs, grabs, and throws toys in play—he does not explore with other types of manipulation. This is one of the early red flags to look for when observing infants and young children who seem slightly hypotonic, are mildly delayed in their gross motor control, and are not playing well, or vocalizing much. These are children whose movement possibilities far exceed the functions they use them for. So this child may pick up a piece of paper and bring it to his mouth using shoulder flexion, elbow and wrist extension for reach, followed by graded elbow flexion with forearm supination. Then, despite the fact that he is 2½ years old, the only thing he does with the paper is stuff it in his mouth, then take it out and tear it to bits. This is what he does with any toy he is given. His upper extremity movements are less graded when he is not looking at what he is doing. His parents tell me that he has destroyed all of his toys and that they are having trouble keeping him in preschool because of complaints of his destructiveness.

I cannot emphasize enough that this is a child with profound disabilities. He may look okay because we see well-developed muscles and a variety of possible movements. He even seems to use his arms the right way (although many people will not notice that he only does so if he is looking at what he is doing). But many times all he does is hit, bite, and throw. So, we erroneously conclude, it must be a behavior problem. After all, he sometimes colors with his crayons, but sometimes just throws or bites them. He is consistently inconsistent, or so it seems. But he is consistent—he only colors when he is looking at the crayons, is not visually distracted by the environment, is seated in a supportive chair, and is given clear, simple instructions with visual guidelines about where to color. Otherwise he throws and bites.

A child with ataxia who is more hypotonic, shows obvious tremors, and has more neuromuscular impairments will be seen as a child who truly has an observable physical disability. This child may show the same behaviors, but her disability will be perceived as a real physical disability, and so is generally better understood and accepted.

Remember that this child's ribcage is rigid and elevated with tight intercostal muscles. This enables the child to belly breathe, possibly combined with use of accessory breathing muscles. Thoracic expansion for deeper, more graded breathing is not possible. In addition, respiration and voicing are not precisely timed (timing is a part of coordination). Together with the probable severe sensory impairments orally, it is not hard to see why many children with ataxia have extremely poor speech. It often is one of their most profound disabilities. In addition, there is the possibility of cognitive deficits, perhaps from the cerebellar lesion itself, that may make speech and language impairments even greater. Finally, remember that many children with ataxia have auditory processing impairments that only add to the impairments already listed.

Functionally, then, limitations result from the altered trunk and ribcage structure, the voluntary holding of the trunk in midline, and the sensory-perceptual impairments. The results are that the child has only a few options for upper extremity function, one option for breathing, and limited trunk movements, primarily in the sagittal plane.

We can look at several children to see the resultant disabilities. A 15-month-old can sit in a variety of positions on the floor, get in and out of sitting independently, creep on all fours, pull to stand, and cruise furniture. She can feed herself Cheerios and drink from a sippy cup independently. She can vocalize "ma" and "ba." In play, however, she grabs, mouths, bites, and throws toys. Rarely does she do anything else.

Occasionally she is seen to pick up something and manipulate it to see it from all sides, then transfer it to the other hand. Her parents report that although she eats well and eats a variety of foods, she only makes two sounds, and often goes for an hour or two without making any sounds.

A 5-year-old learned to walk independently at age 4. He can get in and out of standing independently and is beginning to climb stairs with a handrail. He is extremely cautious in his movement and has to be pushed and coaxed into doing anything new. As he is learning new movements, he cries and clings to his parents and therapists. Once he has mastered the skill he no longer does this, but each time he has to learn another motor skill he goes through the same process. He can feed himself but often mashes finger foods in his hands and doesn't seem to notice. He puts the spoon in his mouth with nothing on it, again not seeming to notice. Although he doesn't throw or bite toys, he does very little in the way of play at all. He sits quietly until he is given structure about what to do. He knows five sign language signs, which he uses to respond to a question from an adult.

A 15-year-old enjoys watching sports on television and watching his older brother play organized sports. His brother often helps him shoot a basketball at home and throw a baseball. The teenager has learned to throw well toward a target when playing one-on-one with his brother. He can feed and dress himself with a strict routine and verbal instructions from his mother. He has many single words that he uses to indicate wants and needs and occasionally puts two or three words together. He cannot write, as his hands tremor too much, and there are cognitive issues as well that prevent him from communicating this way. He cannot manage buttons, snaps, or zippers. He does not tie his shoelaces. His mother describes him as a boy who takes a long time to learn anything new, whether motor or cognitive skills, but that once he learns it, it usually is a part of what he can do. His mother takes him for daily long walks, usually two to three miles. She feels this keeps him in physical shape. She notes that when she first started this that he got short of breath very quickly, but that now he manages quite well and seems to look forward to the walks.

Lower trunk

The child with ataxia shows problems in stability and control of the lower trunk, just as all children with cerebral palsy tend to. In this child there are two major control problems, depending on how the child manages the trunk as a whole. In some children who are more hypotonic and who choose to move very little, being cautious in all they do, the lower trunk functions in a similar way to children with hypotonia. In these children mild thoracic kyphosis is seen in all postures and movements. In the lower trunk the lumbar spine tends to flex into gravity in sitting with decreased hip flexion so that the child tends to sit back on the sacrum. The anterior lower trunk is collapsed so that the sternum and lower ribcage approximate the bony pelvis. The rectus abdominus becomes shortened. This places the weight of the upper body onto the diaphragm and abdominal contents, which forces respiration to become more shallow.

This child may flex the lumbar spine slightly when standing or in prone and on all fours. This may happen when the hip extensors and/or anterior lower trunk musculature (especially the rectus abdominus) shorten over time with habitual posturing. More common, however, is the child who flexes the lumbar spine in sitting, but extends this area when standing. The extension is a passive drop into gravity. The abdominal muscles are still not active in either posture.

There also are a significant number of children with ataxia who are capable of holding their trunks very rigid in extension to prevent weight shifting. These children usually hold the lumbar spine in rigid extension in all postures. The lumbar extensors, especially the erector spinae and the quadratus lumborum, shorten.

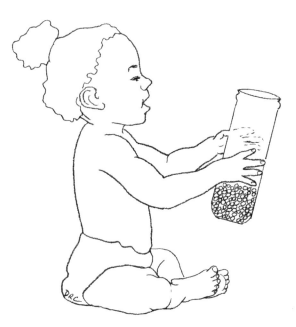

Figure 6.3 This 2-year-old with ataxia can sit, but does not walk. Note her wide lower extremity base of support and strong lumbar extension. This base of support combined with the trunk control she has enables her the proximal control she needs to reach and grasp in space. If she stays in this wide base of support all of the time, however, she will not develop lower trunk and hip control for ambulatory skills.

Although children with ataxia who hold their trunks in rigid extension seem to have better abdominal support for respiration, they still do not use lower trunk flexion, especially with thoracic rotation, to control balance reactions or weight shifting.

Instead, children with ataxia who use rigid trunk extension tend to avoid shifting weight toward the back of their base of support. Often this is accomplished by keeping the upper body forward at all times. Although this compensation enables the child to function in many skills, there are some skills, such as ascending stairs and lower body dressing, that will be difficult to develop because of this. These skills require the child to shift weight posteriorly within the base of support.

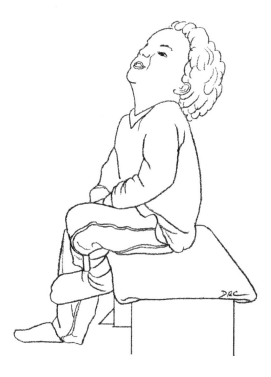

Figure 6.4 This child with ataxia has difficulty lifting his foot up to take his sock off. His legs are strong enough to do this, but he is unwilling to shift his center of mass toward the back of his base of support to take weight off of his legs. Instead he tries to shift weight by extending his cervical spine, which does not move his center of mass. Now he continues to have difficulty lifting his leg and he can no longer see what he is doing.

All children with ataxia, whether excessive flexion or extension is used in the lumbar spine, avoid moving out of a midline posture. Although the child may look as if she is moving the trunk during a function, take a closer look. Most children with ataxia do not move their trunks at all if they can avoid it. Yet they can learn many functions because they can compensate with limb movement in a variety of synergies with joints that are rarely limited in most ranges of motion. As a therapist you must decide whether you can help teach this child a more difficult functional skill without trunk rotation and control of the trunk in all three planes, or whether you must insist that the child incorporate trunk movements into function because the function cannot be learned without it.

The functional limitations, then, result from the limited trunk movements. This is a child who stays in a midline position, whether using lumbar flexion or extension, and avoids movement out of the sagittal plane at all costs. Respiration is impaired in depth because of poor alignment of the ribcage as it connects to the pelvis and because of poor support from abdominal musculature.

Some of the disabilities are as follows: A 2-year-old is able to creep on all fours and pull to stand, cruising along furniture. She stands with her trunk rigidly in extension and increases the stiffness in her lower extremities using cocontraction so that she is usually standing on her toes. She cannot yet walk independently. In sitting, she can use both hands for play as long as there is a table for support of her elbows. Without a table in front of her, she becomes frightened and increases her extension even more. She then refuses to try to use her hands to play. She also starts to gasp for breath.

A 7-year-old who can walk independently is unable to climb stairs without a rail. He also cannot manage curbs or uneven surfaces that are more than 3 inches high. He stays stiffly in extension. He is unable to manage his clothing in dressing and undressing in a standing position and is very slow in dressing when sitting on the floor.

A 13-year-old who uses a wheelchair for mobility is able to talk. Speech is slow and tremorous with little volume. The more fatigued he becomes the more soft his voicing becomes, and he decreases the words per breath he can say. This accompanies an ever more flexed posture of his trunk.

The pelvic girdle and lower extremities

Children with ataxia show two major lower-extremity postures for control of their center of mass. The first relates to those who are more hypotonic and/or who choose to move very little. The child uses a very wide base of support with hips flexed, abducted, and externally rotated; knees usually flexed; and often pronated feet in weight bearing. The child has the mobility to assume this posture and chooses to do so because it provides a wide base of support. The other reason to use this posture, especially hip and knee flexion or hip abduction with flexion, is because it helps lower the center of mass when upright. These are two compensations that many children with ataxia desperately want—a wide base of support and to keep as close to the ground as possible. This way they can be assured that they are more stable. Their tremors, sensory-perceptual impairments, and poor timing of movement all make control against gravity variable and unpredictable for them. So these compensations are an attempt to provide predictability to posture and movement, while at the same time limiting movement that cannot be controlled. A child with ataxia will not give up this compensation easily. Because children with ataxia are so fearful of movement, any attempt to remove predictability of the control that they have learned is rightfully resisted.

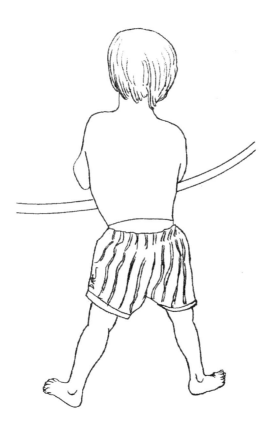

Figure 6.5 This 3-year-old with hypotonia and ataxia is able to pull to stand at furniture. Once standing, he assumes a posture of hip flexion and wide abduction in order to keep his center of mass closer to the ground. However, he is now relatively immobile while in this wide-based stance.

The other major lower-extremity posture in children with ataxia is that they stiffen the lower extremities using voluntary cocontraction. This is a possibility in many children with ataxia, as opposed to many children with athetosis or more severe hypotonia whose neuromuscular impairments prevent the use of cocontraction for any length of time. Children with ataxia may choose this compensation because it is a way to prevent movement in general. It also may be an effective way to dampen tremors. The problem with this compensation is that it prevents the child from using a wide base of support and effectively lowering the center of mass. So in some children, although they stiffen themselves, they actually become more frightened as they then have even less control of their balance. Others may stiffen their lower extremities but assume a posture of hip flexion to keep the center of mass lower, knee hyperextension for joint stability, and ankle plantar flexion.

There are children who manage to stiffen their lower extremities just enough that they can still maintain hip abduction while the hips and knees are almost fully extended. Although this still limits the possibilities of functional skill development, it seems to be the best compensation. It enables many upright skills to develop, although the compensation limits ambulatory skills. There are others who learn to hold with cocontraction in a hip and knee flexed posture to lower their center of mass. The problem with this choice is that the center of mass is now positioned over the back of the base of support, and the child cannot generate enough hip and trunk extension (because he is holding so hard in flexion) to move forward.

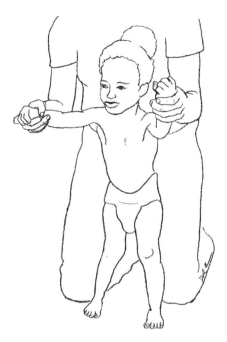

Figure 6.6 The same 2-year-old pictured in Figure 6.3 when supported in standing. She is in hip flexion with abduction, then stiffens herself to assist staying erect. She uses primarily the quadriceps femoris and possibly the hamstrings to stand, but not postural hip extension, so her center of mass stays to the back or behind her base of support.

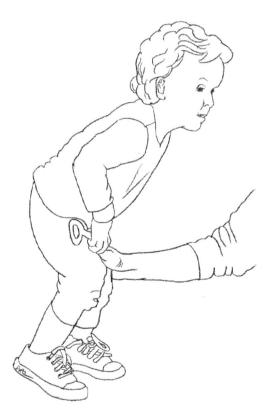

Figure 6.7 This 3-year-old with ataxia and diplegia voluntarily flexes his hips and knees in standing. He verbally expresses fear when placed in standing, and uses the flexion to lower his center of mass. He leans his trunk forward and shifts weight to the front of his feet because the therapist is in front of him. If the therapist moved behind him, he would lean back.

It is easy to see that children with ataxia who use the compensation of excessive cocontraction in the lower extremities to prevent uncontrolled movement are often initially misdiagnosed as children with spastic diplegia. Both use excessive cocontraction, often voluntarily, to control upright postures. Both are very stiff when trying to move them passively. Both can develop joint contractures. However, the child with diplegia is more limited in the use of the synergies she can use in any posture and, unlike the child with ataxia, cannot grade the cocontraction. The child with ataxia, on the other hand, is more sensory impaired, so that giving up a compensation that may provide predictability about where her legs are underneath her is extremely difficult. You may find the child with ataxia more difficult to treat. The child with diplegia is quite willing to use new patterns of movement with more joint range when given to her. The child with ataxia, however, resists attempts at trying to increase weight shifting abilities over more extended and compliant lower extremities. The resistance again is probably due to poor sensory-perceptual awareness of lower extremity position and the unpredictability that results from tremoring and poorly timed movements.

Functional limitations imposed from the movement compensations are a result of using the lower extremities for stability only at the expense of controlled mobility. Whether the child uses a wide base with more passive lower extremity positioning or a narrower base with stiffer legs, the result is that the child is trying to provide stability.

Examples of disabilities include a 2½-year-old who can creep on all fours and pull to stand at very stable furniture, but cannot stand alone or walk. In supported standing at furniture he crouches down and is very stiff. If given support at his trunk by a familiar person who also gets very close to him, he can stand totally erect with properly aligned lower extremities. However, if any attempt is made to decrease the support provided by the adult, he immediately crouches down again. (This is another example of the apparent inconsistency seen in children with ataxia. A casual observer may say that this child can stand up straight if he wants to, so that the child's fears when he crouches are dismissed as uncooperative behavior.)

A 5-year-old can sit, move to all fours, and pull to stand at a weighted, wide-based walker. She cannot walk with the walker without an adult stabilizing it, even with it weighted. She cannot get back down to the floor by herself. She often sits with a very wide base of support on the floor, but when sitting on a bench or chair without armrests, she stiffens herself, especially in the lower body, so that she often falls. Her fears are then confirmed—getting higher against gravity makes her fall.

A 15-year-old who can walk independently can step up some stairs, but not others. People become frustrated with him because it seems that he can step up steps that are high (about 7–9 inches), but refuses to step up lower steps. On careful observation, however, the steps that are lower are more narrow on top with a smaller width and depth than the taller steps, and so provide him less room for a wide-based foot placement as he steps up.

General Treatment Strategies

In treating children with ataxia, your first strategy may be to carefully evaluate how the child uses her eyes. Does she sustain visual gaze on anything? In which visual fields does she seem to sustain that gaze the best? (Children who have motor nystagmus often hold their eyes in the extremes of the periphery of one quadrant to stabilize their gaze). If she does sustain visual gaze, can she then do anything else (shift gaze, shift focal lengths, scan with the head moving, scan with her body moving through space)? Usually there is a breakdown of abilities somewhere.

Take a child who has established no consistent visual attention into a small, uncluttered room with a chair and one toy or book and begin treatment in this environment. Combine correct sitting or standing alignment with insistence on visual attention on something that the child is most likely to look at. This can be extremely difficult and tedious work. Success sometimes is measured in the number of seconds the child sustains gaze or the small number of times the child visually focuses in a given time period. When working with children with ataxia you must be extremely organized (almost to a ritual at first) and repetitious, with only one to two activities to get any results. Treatment, therefore, can be difficult and trying for everyone involved. Yet this establishment of visual attention and sustained visual gaze is imperative to success.

Once the child looks at something, she begins to be able to use visual stability to help stabilize more postures and movement through space. There often can be a dramatic difference in the ability to hold postures and grade movements once visual attention is gained. Treatment then becomes very rewarding. Progress to having the child maintain a stable posture, often sitting, while shifting her gaze and leading head movement with eye movement to search for something. Ask the child to use downward visual gaze while in a stable position, which always seems the most difficult. Ask for the same head and eye movements when the child is moving through space. Of course, this sequence can be entered into wherever the child needs to start.

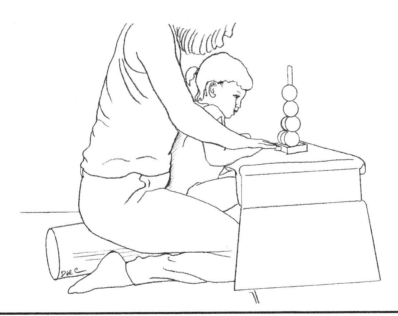

Figure 6.8   As this child is asked to look down at a toy, her therapist contacts the child's body with her own body. She also gives her firm pressure into the support surface. This overall firm contact may reassure the child proprioceptively and tactilely about body position in space. She is then more willing to use her eyes for movement and gaze downward.

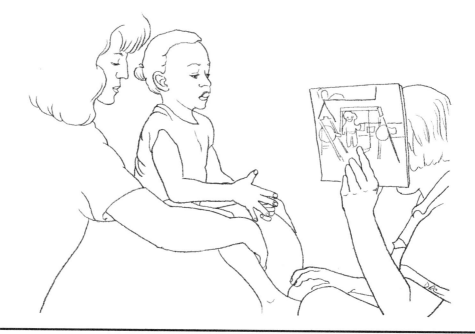

Figure 6.9 Once firmly seated and supported, this child is willing to shift her gaze from looking straight ahead to down. Her therapist may play a game with her to increase the speed at which she can shift her gaze.

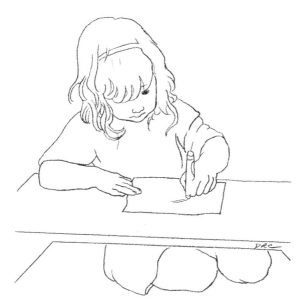

Figure 6.10 This child can now shift her eyes and use head flexion on her cervical spine on her own as she colors. However, she must be positioned close to the floor with a wide base of support to do this. She does not look down when she is walking.

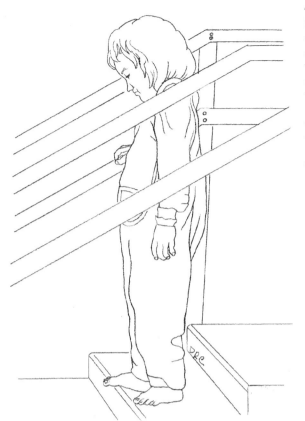

Figure 6.11 This 6-year-old with ataxia is able to look down as she descends the staircase. This was not an easy skill for her to learn. Her therapists tried a variety of techniques to help her learn to shift her gaze down with only partial success. They tried joint approximation through a well-aligned spine and lower extremities, painting her toenails to encourage sustained downward visual gaze, and practice with repetition. The technique that finally worked well was to give her oral control (as shown in Figure 5.44) while she descended the stairs. The firm contact with her oral area seemed to focus her attention and make her secure with the movement of downward visual gaze. After several repetitions within one session, she was able to descend the stairs on her own using downward visual gaze.

Visual attention is combined with movement (as stated previously) when the child is able to handle both. Work to establish correct midline postures, which is usually relatively easy since children with ataxia like to be in midline. But then you must move out and away from midline. This again can be a very difficult part of treatment and extremely frightening to the child. This fear on the child's part comes as no surprise to anyone who works with a child who has always been cautious and fearful. What can be surprising is that the same experience will be just as frightening to the child who always seems to be running everywhere. Yet this child will have the same problem of holding herself stiffly in midline and not wanting to be moved out of this position.

Because moving away from midline is so frightening to the child, consider whether it is necessary that the child learns to move out of midline to achieve the functional goal. If the answer is yes, then use gentle, firm insistence that movements away from midline occur. If the answer is no, then there is no reason to push the child into a fearful situation. If you do decide that the child needs to make a movement that creates fear, work to keep the child physically close to you at first. Perform the movement with him. Give him deep pressure by handling him firmly during the movement, even though motorically he may not need to be handled so much. Your handling offers sensory-perceptual input that provides security for the child.

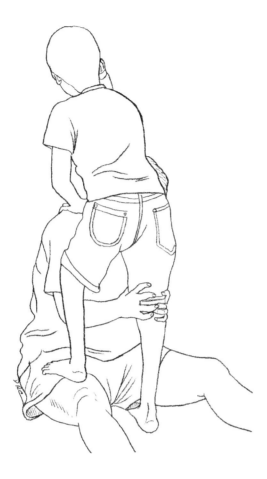

Figure 6.12 This child is learning to climb stairs with one hand on the rail. He is very frightened of shifting his weight onto one leg as he lifts the other, and so cannot complete the skill. His therapist works in front of him so that the child can see her. She keeps close to him and allows him to contact her with his hands and one foot. As she helps him shift weight onto one foot, she leans her body in the direction of that foot.

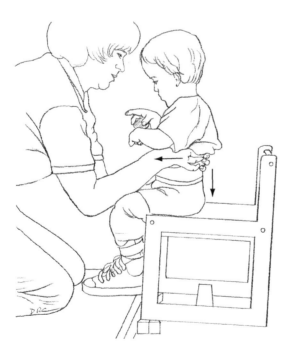

Figure 6.13 This child's speech pathologist works to first help him extend his trunk. She then will rotate his trunk as he speaks to help him prolong exhalation. She also may use manual vibration as a treatment technique while she rotates his trunk to help him prolong the exhalation.

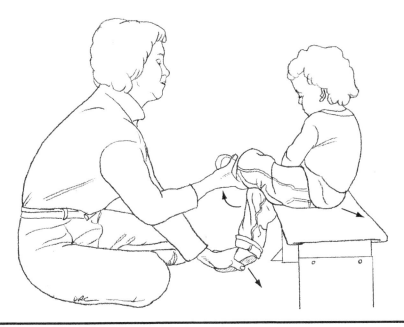

Figure 6.14 This child from Figure 6.4 is now helped to lift his foot to take off his sock. His therapist assists him to keep his right foot on the floor while assisting flexion and external rotation of the other hip. She also shifts his weight toward the back of his base of support, the most difficult part of the posture and movement for this child. If he becomes frightened, as he used to several months ago, his therapist would move closer to him and probably support his lower trunk with one of her hands.

In treating a child with ataxia, it is likely that any movement or function that you teach her will be entirely new to her. Textbooks say that the cerebellum has a large responsibility in motor learning and probably in learning in general, and clinical experience confirms it. Therefore, you may find little to no use for simulation activities in treatment—games that are *like* the function, but are not the function itself. To a child with ataxia, nothing is like anything else. If you want the child to learn to drink out of a cup, then ask his parents to bring his cup if you will not see him at his home. When drinking from this cup is established, do not be surprised if the child can only drink from this one cup. He may then have to learn how to drink out of other cups. You also may find, unfortunately, that children with ataxia have good and bad days. One day they seem to know or have learned something, and the next it may not be part of what they can do. Again assume this has something to do with the impairments in learning caused by the lesion. This applies to motor learning as well as classroom learning as reported by teachers.

The tremendous difficulties that children with ataxia have in learning can be frustrating and overwhelming. You cannot imagine how frustrating it must be for the child and his family. Because children with ataxia have great difficulty learning new motor skills, they often are more severely involved functionally than they initially appear. This is why children with ataxia are every bit as disabled as other children with cerebral palsy, sometimes more so. Although at first impression they may seem more mildly involved because their alignment, muscle bulk, strength, and variety of movements are not as impaired as those of children with hypertonia, hypotonia, and athetosis, their sensory-perceptual and learning impairments may be so severe that new skill acquisition is extremely difficult.

Finally, children with ataxia require a great amount of advocacy and family support in addition to what you usually may do for children with cerebral palsy. This is because you must spend a great deal of time explaining the child's disability to people with whom the child interacts and confirming for the family that the child has real and profound sensory motor impairments, not just an undetermined behavioral problem. In addition, you often must teach the child, his family, and the community about how to keep the child and others safe in their environments—others because the child approaches them too forcefully, and the child himself because he does not use sensory systems well to monitor movement through space.

CASE STUDY

To conclude, look at two children with ataxia and follow a treatment sequence toward a functional goal. The first is a young child of 18 months who is just learning to walk independently. She cannot yet run or stand up from the middle of the floor. She cannot stand still—she always seems to be dancing in place if she is not walking. She can feed herself finger foods and is starting to use a fork after her parents stab the food for her. She makes two sounds—"ba" and "ma." Her family wants her to learn to stand still so that they can begin dressing her in standing and so she can stop while walking and reach for toys on the floor. Her mother is concerned that if her child cannot learn to stand still that this will cause problems in group activities when she goes to preschool. As the child's physical therapist, your plan may be to first look at her visual skills in standing. You may see that she is a child who looks at a target across a room and walks toward it. She does not visually scan the room, and often trips and falls on any object in her path. Remember that it is not uncommon for 18-month-olds to not watch where they are going and to trip and fall on objects in their paths. But most 18-month-olds developing normally are perfectly capable of standing still. Look to see if she ever shifts her eyes downward toward her feet while she stands. She does not. Children developing normally frequently look at their feet while standing and look down prior to squatting to the floor to retrieve a dropped toy.

Begin treatment in sitting because she probably will not be as fearful in shifting her gaze in a more supported posture that she has more experience with. Use a book, toy, or your voice to gain visual attention and to help her sustain it. You may use joint approximation through a well-aligned spine in sitting and through the ankles to help her sit still and to be more aware proprioceptively of her posture. Give her firm muscle proprioceptive and tactile input at her hips and thighs into the chair she is sitting on to help her become more aware of her base of support. Slowly lead her visual gaze to the lower quadrants until she begins to lead head movement with downward visual gaze. Then ask her to stand up and hold a toy as she looks at it. Get very close to her and hold her against you, even though motorically she does not need this much support. Go through the same visual routine again in standing. Begin to ask her to look down prior to picking up a toy from the floor. Help her keep her postural control with deep pressure and joint approximation to help her not be so fearful that she will not risk looking down. After she is able to pick up a toy from the floor by first visually locating it, then ask her to hold the toy as she stands and continues to look at it. It is through this visual attention that she first learns to stand still.

As a home program, ask her parents to encourage their daughter to look directly at body parts being dressed. Her parents are to name the part of the body going into or out of clothing and encourage her to look. Suggest that they rub her skin briskly and firmly to call her visual attention to the body area. When her pants are placed over her feet and around her ankles, her parents will place her in a standing position and ask her to look down, then reach down to assist pulling up her pants.

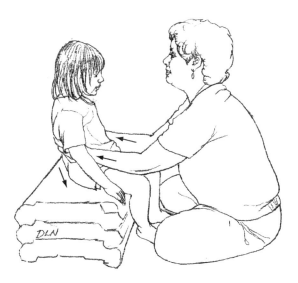

Figure 6.15 The therapist shows this child's mother how to support the child's lower ribcage to maintain thoracic extension while tilting her slightly back toward the back edge of her base of support. Tilting the child back facilitates a chin tuck and helps the child look straight ahead or slightly downward instead of using her typical upward visual gaze. In this way, the child is prepared to look at her own body while assisting dressing.

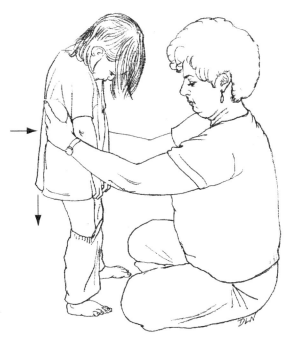

Figure 6.16 After using this home program for assisted dressing for several weeks, the therapist next shows the child's mother how to support the child's ribcage in the same place while keeping her in thoracic extension. The therapist's or mother's hands can then also push firmly and repetitively toward the ground to give somatosensory information to the child about her body position while standing. The child is then asked to look and reach down to pull up her pants.

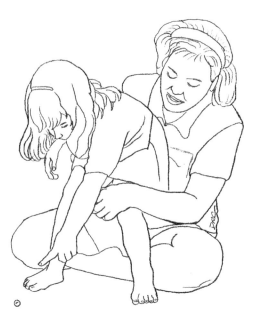

Figure 6.17 A fun way to practice looking down while moving in standing is to follow and pop bubbles. This child's mother supports her as she reaches and looks down.

As the child's speech pathologist, you will evaluate language skills as well as the sensorimotor skills. In looking specifically at the latter, you may decide that this child is capable of making more sounds than she is currently using. Evaluate her breath support for this as well as her oral motor skills. You note that her breathing is rapid and shallow, with a belly-breathing pattern. She also does not move her tongue separately from her jaw. She has difficulty grading her jaw movement for speech sound production. The timing of the downward excursion of the jaw is longer than it should be. The lack of timing and precision impacts on both correct articulatory postures and on resonance. She uses atypical oral movements of the lips and cheeks with tongue retraction as an attempt to stabilize her body posture while doing many functional activities. This includes feeding, speech, and swallowing as well as many other gross and fine motor activities.

In treatment, assist her first to sustain active trunk posture and movements in all three planes. Ensure that she uses enough thoracic extension and control of rotation to support longer and more controlled exhalation. The more active stability in her trunk also reduces her need for the atypical oral movements and the tongue retraction. Next you can use the inhibitory technique of manual vibration on the cheeks and at the base of the tongue to assist the facial and tongue muscles to terminate the sustained retracted postures. Ask for graded jaw movements through repeated biting activities to assist with more rapid and precise timing of jaw movements. Finally, ask for the particular sound desired as she imitates you. Insist on visual attention and also ask her to touch your face as you make the sound (as a way to assist visual attention and as way to give organized, meaningful, multisensory systems information for learning). Ask her parents to do this last activity, too—they can help their daughter touch their faces as they encourage her to look directly at them at selected times of the day. They may find that mealtime in her highchair or bath time is a good time to practice looking and touching their faces as they say particular words.

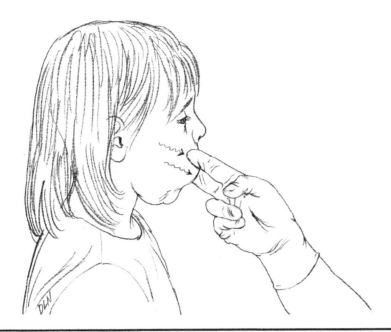

Figure 6.18 Manual vibration is used on the child to help her terminate contraction of sustained retraction of her lips and cheeks. One finger is placed inside the child's cheek and the other on the outside of her cheek. As the soft tissue is vibrated, the cheek is gently pulled toward midline as the therapist's finger slowly is removed from inside her mouth.

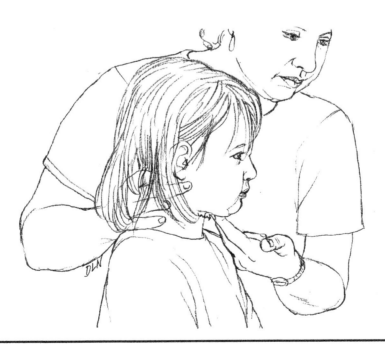

Figure 6.19 Manual vibration also is used to bring the tongue out of its retracted position. The therapist supports the child's head position with one hand and vibrates on the outside of the child's jaw at the base of her tongue, lifting the tongue and moving it forward.

The second child is a 13-year-old who uses a wheelchair for mobility. He does not walk independently, but can walk if an adult holds one of his arms. This teenager is able to propel his wheelchair manually for short, classroom distances but is very slow. He is able to speak in phrases in a very monotone voice with a slow pace. It takes him a long time to say what he wants to say. He seems to stare at the person he speaks to or to stare at something in the room. When he is asked to look at something else, he slowly shifts his gaze, then stares at the next object. He can do some self-dressing, but cannot put on his outdoor coat, pull up his trousers and zip them, or put on shoes and socks. His teacher has asked his consulting occupational therapist to help find a way for him to put on his coat to go home in the afternoons.

You may have the advantage of seeing this child in a real situation with his own coat. He sits in his classroom chair to put on his coat. After watching him attempt the task, you may see that as soon as the coat is out of his visual field, he performs much worse. In addition, he does not try to move his head or trunk to visually search for the sleeve of the coat when he loses sight of it. He also does not rotate his trunk to assist his reach nor does he move his arms overhead away from his trunk to push them through the sleeves.

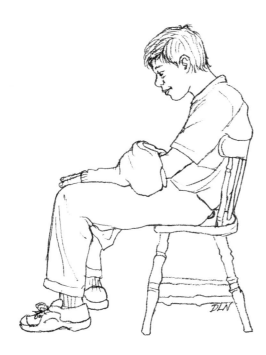

Figure 6.20 This teenager sits in a classroom chair that is small for his height. He is likely to feel unsafe when moving. As soon as he begins to attempt to lift his arms away from his lap, he becomes fearful. In addition, in this chair he is unwilling or unable to actively extend or rotate his spine. He will probably need one or both of these movements in order to be successful in putting on his coat.

Because you are a consulting therapist who sees this young man once a month, you must ask his teacher and aide to perform the direct intervention. Remember to be knowledgeable about the daily classroom routine and the heavy demands placed upon the teacher's and aide's time each day. If your instructions fit into the routine they already have to do, the classroom program is much more likely to get done. You may suggest that when helping the young man to put on his coat, he should first sit in his wheelchair because it is more supportive and he uses it on the bus trip home. The teacher could ask him to look at his arm as he raises it or is assisted in raising it. She then should hold his arm firmly, perhaps vigorously rubbing it to help him feel its position. She should wait for him to process the request of lifting up his arm, giving him time to respond.

You may entirely alter the way he puts on his coat and teach this to the teacher and aide. You may select a way that enables the young man to stay more in midline and keep the coat in front of him longer so that he can see it longer. He could put both arms in first as the jacket lays on his lap, then lift both arms overhead to put on the jacket. This would enable him to avoid trunk rotation and to see the jacket longer, but would require at least brief thoracic and lumbar extension as both arms reach overhead.

You also may want to evaluate the support that the wheelchair provides or movements that the wheelchair allows or does not allow. Changes to the seating system may enable the young man to be more secure in sitting so that he is more willing to turn his head, look down, or rotate his trunk if he is capable of these movements.

There are probably other options that you can think of. Just keep in mind the role of the teacher and aide (they assist with coats at the end of a day, but are not trained to do stretching exercises, trunk control issues, and so forth). Keep in mind the easiest ways to teach this skill given the impairments that you observe interfering with the task, such as keeping the coat close to the adolescent, teaching him to look at it, placing it in a position where he can see it most of the time, and using movement strategies that allow him to feel safe within his base of support. Be open to feedback from the teacher and aide—both positive and negative. If your instruction doesn't work, you will want to know this and try another way.

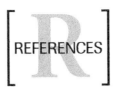

REFERENCES

Agnarsson, U., Warde, C., McCarthy, G., Clayden, G. S., & Evans, N. (1993). Anorectal function of children with neurological problems: II. Cerebral palsy. *Developmental Medicine and Child Neurology, 35,* 903–908.

Albright, A. L., Cervi, A., & Singletary, J. (1991). Intrathecal baclofen for spasticity in cerebral palsy. *Journal of the American Medical Association, 265*(11), 1418–1422.

Alexander, R., Boehme, R., & Cupps, B. (1993). *Normal development of functional motor skills.* San Antonio, TX: Therapy Skill Builders.

Almeida, G. L., Corcos, D. M., & Latash, M. L. (1994). Practice and transfer effects during fast single-joint elbow movements in individuals with Down syndrome. *Physical Therapy, 74*(11), 1000–1016.

American Academy for Cerebral Palsy and Developmental Medicine. (1996). *The history of the American Academy for Cerebral Palsy and Developmental Medicine.* Rosemont, IL: Author.

Arnold, A. S., Komattu, A. V., & Delp, S. L. (1997). Internal rotation gait: A compensatory mechanism to restore abduction capacity decreased by bone deformity? *Developmental Medicine and Child Neurology, 39,* 40–44.

Aronsson, D. D., Stokes, I. A. F., Ronchetti, P. J., & Labelle, H. B. (1994). Comparison of curve shape between children with cerebral palsy, Friedreich's ataxia, and adolescent idiopathic scoliosis. *Developmental Medicine and Child Neurology, 36,* 412–418.

Bastian, A. J. (1997). Mechanisms of ataxia. *Physical Therapy, 77*(6), 672–675.

Bartlett, D., & Piper, M. C. (1993). Neuromotor development of preterm infants through the first year of life: Implications for physical and occupational therapists. *Physical and Occupational Therapy in Pediatrics, 12*(4), 37–55.

Berger, W., Quintern, J., & Dietz, V. (1982). Pathophysiology of gait in children with cerebral palsy. *Electroencephalography and Clinical Neurophysiology, 53,* 538–548.

Bertenthal, B. I., & Campos, J. J. (1987). New directions in the study of early experience. *Child Development, 58,* 560–567.

Blair, E., Ballantyne, J., Horsman, S., & Chauvel, P. (1995). A study of a dynamic proximal stability splint in the management of children with cerebral palsy. *Developmental Medicine and Child Neurology, 37,* 544–554.

Bly, L. (1994). *Motor skills acquisition in the first year: An illustrated guide to normal development.* San Antonio, TX: Therapy Skill Builders.

Bobath, K. (1971). The normal postural reflex mechanism and its deviation in children with cerebral palsy. *Physiotherapy, 57,* 515–525.

Bobath, B. (1971). Motor development, its effect on general development, and application to the treatment of cerebral palsy. *Physiotherapy, 57,* 526–532.

Bobath, B. (1985). *Abnormal postural reflex activity caused by brain lesion* (3rd ed.). Oxford: Butterworth-Heinemann.

Bobath, K., & Bobath, B. (1964). The facilitation of normal postural reactions and movements in the treatment of cerebral palsy. *Physiotherapy, 50,* 246–262.

Bobath, K., & Bobath, B. (1972). Cerebral palsy. In P. H. Pearson and C. E. Williams (Eds.), *Physical therapy services in the developmental disabilities* (pp. 31–185). Springfield, IL: Charles C. Thomas.

Bobath, B., & Bobath, K. (1975). *Motor development in the different types of cerebral palsy.* Oxford: Heinemann Medical Books.

Boiteau, M., Malouin, F., & Richards, C. L. (1995). Use of a hand-held dynamometer and a Kin-Com dynamometer for evaluating spastic hypertonia in children: A reliability study. *Physical Therapy, 75*(9), 796–802.

Borzyskowski, M. (1989). Cerebral palsy and the bladder. *Developmental Medicine and Child Neurology, 31,* 687–689.

Bradley, N. (1994). Motor control: Developmental aspects of motor control in skill acquisition. In S. Campbell (Ed.), *Physical therapy for children* (pp. 45–46). Philadelphia: W. B. Saunders.

Brashear, H. R., & Raney, R. B. (1978). Affections of the spine and thorax. In A. R. Shands (Ed.), *Handbook of Orthopaedic Surgery* (9th ed.) (pp. 313–332). St. Louis: C. V. Mosby.

Brogren, E., Hadders-Algra, M., & Forssberg, H. (1996). Postural control in children with spastic diplegia: Muscle activity during perturbations in sitting. *Developmental Medicine and Child Neurology, 38,* 379–388.

Brown, J. K. (Ed.). (1993). Science and spasticity. *Developmental Medicine and Child Neurology, 35,* 471–472.

Butterworth, G., & Hicks, L. (1977). Visual proprioception and postural stability in infancy: A developmental study. *Perception, 6,* 255–262.

Carey, J. R., & Burghardt, T. P. (1993). Movement dysfunction following central nervous system lesions: A problem of neurologic or muscular impairment? *Physical Therapy, 73*(8), 538–547.

Carmick, J. (1995a). Managing equinus in a child with cerebral palsy: Merits of hinged ankle-foot orthoses. *Developmental Medicine and Child Neurology, 37,* 1006–1010.

Carmick, J. (1995b). Managing equinus in children with cerebral palsy: Electrical stimulation to strengthen the triceps surae muscle. *Developmental Medicine and Child Neurology, 37,* 965–975.

Cassidy, C., Craig, C. L., Perry, A., Karlin, L. I., & Goldberg M. J. (1994). A reassessment of spinal stabilization in severe cerebral palsy. *Journal of Pediatric Orthopaedics, 14,* 731–739.

Castle, M. E., Reyman, T. A., & Schneider, M. (1979). Pathology of spastic muscle in cerebral palsy. *Clinical Orthopedics and Related Research, 142,* 223–233.

Chauvel, P. J., Horsman, S., Ballantyne, J., & Blair, E. (1993). Lycra splinting and the management of cerebral palsy. *Developmental Medicine and Child Neurology, 35,* 456–459.

Cioni, G., Fazzi, B., Ipata, A. E., Canapicchi, R., & van Hof-van Duin, J. (1996). Correlation between cerebral visual impairment and magnetic resonance imaging in children with neonatal encephalopathy. *Developmental Medicine and Child Neurology, 38,* 120–132.

Cole, K. J., Abbs, J. H., & Turner, G. S. (1988). Deficits in the production of grip forces in Down syndrome. *Developmental Medicine and Child Neurology, 30,* 752–758.

Coniglio, S. J., Stevenson, R. D., & Rogol, A. D. (1996). Apparent growth hormone deficiency in children with cerebral palsy. *Developmental Medicine and Child Neurology, 38,* 797–804.

Conroy, J. (Director). (1990). *My left foot* [Videotape]. Toronto: Cineplex Odeon Corporation.

Coon, V., Donato, G., Houser, C., & Bleck, E. E. (1975). Normal ranges of hip motion in infants 6 weeks, 3 months, and 6 months of age. *Clinical Orthopaedics and Related Research, 110,* 256–260.

Cornell, M. S. (1995). The hip in cerebral palsy. *Developmental Medicine and Child Neurology, 37,* 3–18.

Crawford, C. L., & Hobbs, M. J. (1994). Anatomy of diplegia: An hypothesis. *Developmental Medicine and Child Neurology, 36,* 513–517.

Damiano, D. L. (1993). Reviewing muscle cocontraction: Is it a developmental, pathological, or motor control issue? *Physical and Occupational Therapy in Pediatrics, 12*(4), 3–20.

Davis, W. E., & Kelso, J. A. S. (1982). Analysis of "invariant characteristics" in the motor control of Down's syndrome and normal subjects. *Journal of Motor Behavior, 14*(3), 194–212.

Deford, F. (1997). *Alex: The life of a child.* Nashville, TN: Rutledge Hill Press.

Diamond, L. S., Lynne, D., & Sigman, B. (1981). Orthopedic disorders in patients with Down's syndrome. *Orthopedic Clinics of North America, 12*(1), 57–71.

Dietz, V., & Berger, W. (1995). Cerebral palsy and muscle transformation. *Developmental Medicine and Child Neurology, 37*, 180–184.

Dofferhof, A. S. M., & Vink, P. (1985). The stabilizing function of the mm. iliocostales and the mm. multifidi during walking. *Journal of Anatomy, 140*(2), 329–336.

Dorland's Illustrated Medical Dictionary (28th ed.). (1984). Philadelphia: W. B. Saunders.

Doyon, J. (1997). Skill learning. *International Review of Neurobiology, 41*, 273–294.

Duckman, R. H. (1979). The incidence of visual anomalies in a population of cerebral palsied children. *Journal of the American Optometric Association 50*(9), 1013–1016.

Duckman, R. H. (1984). Accommodation in cerebral palsy: Function and remediation. *Journal of the American Optometric Association, 55*(4), 281–283.

Duckman, R. H. 1987. Vision therapy for the child with cerebral palsy. *Journal of the American Optometric Association, 58*(1), 28–35.

Eliasson, A. C., Gordon, A. M., & Forssberg, H. (1991). Basic co-ordination of manipulative forces of children with cerebral palsy. *Developmental Medicine and Child Neurology, 33*, 661–670.

Eliasson, A. C., Gordon, A. M., & Forssberg, H. (1992). Impaired anticipatory control of isometric forces during grasping by children with cerebral palsy. *Developmental Medicine and Child Neurology, 34*, 216–225.

Esscher, E., Flodmark, O., Hagberg, G., & Hagberg, B. (1996). Non-progressive ataxia: Origins, brain pathology and impairments in 78 Swedish children. *Developmental Medicine and Child Neurology, 38*, 285–296.

Fenichel, G. M. (1982). The newborn with poor muscle tone. *Seminars in Perinatology, 6*(1), 68–88.

Foley, J. (1983). The athetoid syndrome: A review of a personal series. *Journal of Neurology, Neurosurgery, and Psychiatry, 46*, 289–298.

Foley, J., (1992). Dyskinetic and dystonic cerebral palsy and birth. *Acta Paediatrica Scandinavica, 81*, 57–60.

Fuji, T., Yonenobu, K., Fujiwara, K., Yamashita, K., Ebara, S., Ono, K., & Okada, K. (1987). Cervical radiculopathy or myelopathy secondary to athetoid cerebral palsy. *The Journal of Bone and Joint Surgery, 69-A*(6), 815–821.

Gage, J. R. (1991). *Gait analysis in cerebral palsy.* (Clinics in Developmental Medicine, No.121). New York: Cambridge University.

Gajdosik, C. G., & Ostertag, S. (1996). Cervical instability and Down syndrome: Review of the literature and implications for physical therapists. *Pediatric Physical Therapy, 8*, 31–36.

Goodman, R., & Yude, C. (1996). IQ and its predictors in childhood hemiplegia. *Developmental Medicine and Child Neurology, 38*, 881–890.

Gordon, J. (1987). Assumptions underlying physical therapy intervention: Theoretical and historical perspectives. In J. H. Carr & R. B. Shepherd (Eds.), *Movement sciences: Foundations for physical therapy in rehabilitation* (pp. 1–30). Rockville, MD: Aspen Systems.

Haas, S. S., Epps, C. H., & Adams, J. P. (1973). Normal ranges of hip motion in the newborn. *Clinical Orthopaedics and Related Research, 91*, 114–118.

Hadders-Algra, M. A., Bos, F., Martijn, A., & Prechtl, H. F. R. (1994). Infantile chorea in an infant with severe bronchopulmonary dysplasia: An EMG study. *Developmental Medicine and Child Neurology, 36,* 173–182.

Hagberg, B., & Hagberg, G. (1992). Invited commentary: Dyskinetic and dystonic cerebral palsy and birth. *Acta Paediatrica Scandinavica, 81,* 93–94.

Hainsworth, F., Harrison, M. J., Sheldon, T. A., & Roussounis, S. H. (1997). A preliminary evaluation of ankle orthoses in the management of children with cerebral palsy. *Developmental Medicine and Child Neurology, 39,* 243–247.

Hallett, M., & Alvarez, N. (1983). Attempted rapid elbow flexion movements in patients with athetosis. *Journal of Neurology, Neurosurgery, and Psychiatry, 46,* 745–750.

Hallett, M., & Grafman, J. (1997). Executive function and motor skill learning. *International Review of Neurobiology, 41,* 297–223.

Hallett, M., Shahani, B. T., & Young, R. R. (1975). EMG analysis of patients with cerebellar deficits. *Journal of Neurology, Neurosurgery, and Psychiatry, 38,* 1163–1169.

Harada, T., Ebara, S., Anwar, M. M., Kajiura, I., Oshita, S., Hiroshima, K., & Ono, K. (1993). The lumbar spine in spastic diplegia. *The Journal of Bone and Joint Surgery, 75-B,* 534–537.

Harada, T., Ebara, S., Anwar, M. M., Okawa, A., Kajiura, I., Hiroshima, K., & Ono, K. (1996). The cervical spine in athetoid cerebral palsy. *The Journal of Bone and Joint Surgery, 78*(4), 613–619.

Hebbandi, S. B., Bowen, J. R., Hipwell, G. C., Ma, D. J., Leslie, G. I., & Arnold, J. D. (1997). Ocular sequelae in extremely premature infants at 5 years of age. *Journal of Paediatrics and Child Health, 33,* 339–342.

Heine, R. G., Reddihough, D. S., & Catto-Smith, A. G. (1995). Gastro-oesophageal reflux and feeding problems after gastrostomy in children with severe neurological impairment. *Devlopmental Medicine and Child Neurology, 37,* 320–329.

Held, R. (1965). Plasticity in sensory-motor systems. *Scientific American, 213*(5), 84–95.

Hodges, P. W., & Richardson, C. A. (1997). Contraction of the abdominal muscles associated with movement of the lower limb. *Physical Therapy, 77*(2), 132–144.

Ito, J., Saijo, H., Araki, A., Tanaka, H., Tasaki, T., Cho, K., & Miyamoto, A. (1996). Assessment of visuoperceptual disturbance in children with spastic diplegia using measurements of the lateral ventricles on cerebral MRI. *Developmental Medicine and Child Neurology, 38,* 496–502.

Janda, V. (1978). Muscles, central nervous motor regulation, and back problems. In I. M. Korr (Ed.), *The neurobiologic mechanisms in manipulative therapy (pp. 27–41).* New York: Plenum Press.

Jette, A. M. (1995). Outcomes research: Shifting the dominant research paradigm in physical therapy. *Physical Therapy, 75*(11), 965–970.

Johnson, R. K., Goran, M. I., Ferrara, M. S., & Poehlman, E. T. (1996). Athetosis increases resting metabolic rate in adults with cerebral palsy. *Journal of the American Dietetic Association, 96*(2), 145–148.

Kelly, M. K. (1994). Children with ventilator dependence. In S. Campbell (Ed.), *Physical Therapy for Children* (pp. 663–685). Philadelphia: W. B. Saunders Company.

Krebs, D. E., Wong, D., Jevsevar, D., Riley, P. O., & Hodge, W. A. (1992). Trunk kinematics during locomotor activities. *Physical Therapy, 72*(7), 505–514.

Kuban, K. C. K. & Leviton, A. (1994). Cerebral palsy. *The New England Journal of Medicine, 330*(3), 188–195.

Laplaza, F. J., & Root, L. (1994). Femoral anteversion and neck-shaft angles in hip instability in cerebral palsy. *Journal of Pediatric Orthopaedics, 14,* 719–723.

Lee, W. (1984). Neuromotor synergies as a basis for coordinated intentional action. *Journal of Motor Behavior, 16*(2), 135–170.

Lee, W. A. (1988). A control systems framework for understanding normal and abnormal posture. *The American Journal of Occupational Therapy, 43*(5), 291–301.

Lee, D. N., & Aronson, E. (1974). Visual proprioceptive control of standing in human infants. *Perception and Psychophysics, 15*(3), 529–532.

Leonard, C. T., Hirschfeld, H., & Forssberg, H. (1991). The development of independent walking in children with cerebral palsy. *Developmental Medicine and Child Neurology, 33,* 567–577.

LeVeau, B. F., & Bernhardt, D. B. (1984). Developmental biomechanics: Effect of forces on the growth, development, and maintenance of the human body. *Physical Therapy, 64*(12), 1874–1882.

Levitt, S. (1995). *Treatment of cerebral palsy and motor delay.* (3rd ed.) Cambridge, MA: Blackwell Science Ltd.

Lin, J. P., Brown, J. K., & Brotherstone, R. (1994). Assessment of spasticity in hemiplegic cerebral palsy: II. Distal lower-limb reflex excitability and function. *Developmental Medicine and Child Neurology, 36,* 290–303.

Lin, P. P., & Henderson, R. C. (1996). Bone mineralization in the affected extremities of children with spastic hemiplegia. *Developmental Medicine and Child Neurology, 38,* 782–786.

Mandich, M. B., Simons, C. J. R., Ritchie, S., Schmidt, D., & Mullett, M. (1994). Motor development, infantile reactions, and postural responses of preterm, at-risk infants. *Developmental Medicine and Child Neurology, 36,* 397–405.

Miedaner, J. A., & Renander, J. (1987). The effectiveness of classroom passive stretching programs for increasing or maintaining passive range of motion in non-ambulatory children: An evaluation of frequency. *Physical and Occupational Therapy in Pediatrics, 7*(3), 35–43.

Miller, G. (1989). Minor congenital anomalies and ataxic cerebral palsy. *Archives of Disease in Childhood, 64,* 557–562.

Mossberg, K. A., Linton, K. A., & Friske, K. (1990). Ankle-foot orthoses: Effect on energy expenditure of gait in spastic diplegic children. *Archives of Physical Medicine and Rehabilitation, 71,* 490–494.

Nashner, L. M., Shumway-Cook, A., & Marin, O. (1983). Stance posture control in select groups of children with cerebral palsy: Deficits in sensory organization and muscular coordination. *Experimental Brain Research, 49,* 393–409.

Newton, P. M. (1995). *Freud: From youthful dream to midlife crisis.* New York: The Guilford Press.

Olney, S. J., & Wright, M. J. (1994). Cerebral palsy. In S. K. Campbell (Ed.), *Physical Therapy for Children* (pp. 489–492, 498–499, 513). Philadelphia: W. B. Saunders Company.

Opila-Lehman, J., Short, M. A., & Trombly, C. A. (1985). Kinesthetic recall of children with athetoid and spastic cerebral palsy and of non-handicapped children. *Developmental Medicine and Child Neurology, 27,* 223–230.

O'Shea, T. M., Goldstein, D. J., deRegnier, R. A., Sheaffer, C. I., Roberts, D. D., & Dillard, R. G. (1996). Outcome at 4 to 5 years of age in children recovered from neonatal chronic lung disease. *Developmental Medicine and Child Neurology, 38,* 830–839.

Ostrosky, K. M. (1990). Facilitation vs. motor control. *Clinical Management, 10*(3), 34–40.

Parker, D. F., Carriere, L., Hebestreit, H., & Salsberg, A., & Bar-Or, O. (1993). Muscle performance and gross motor function of children with spastic cerebral palsy. *Developmental Medicine and Child Neurology, 35,* 17–23.

Perry, J. (1992). *Gait analysis: Normal and pathological function.* Thorofare, NJ: Slack.

Perry, J., Antonelli, D., & Ford, W. (1975). Analysis of knee-joint forces during flexed-knee stance. *The Journal of Bone and Joint Surgery, 57-A*(7), 961–967.

Perry, J., Hoffer, M. M., Giovan, P., Antonelli, D., & Greenberg, R. (1974). Gait analysis of the triceps surae in cerebral palsy. *The Journal of Bone and Joint Surgery, 56-A*(3), 511–520.

Pimentel, E. D. (1996). The disappearing reflex: A reevaluation of its role in normal and abnormal development. *Physical and Occupational Therapy in Pediatrics, 16*(4), 19–41.

Pope, D. F., Bueff, H. U., & DeLuca, P. A. (1994). Pelvic osteotomies for subluxation of the hip in cerebral palsy. *Journal of Pediatric Orthopaedics, 14,* 724–730.

Radtka, S. A., Skinner, S. R., Dixon, D. M., & Johanson, M. E. (1997). A comparison of gait with solid, dynamic, and no ankle-foot orthoses in children with spastic cerebral palsy. *Physical Therapy, 77*(4), 395–409.

Reese, M. E., Msall, M. E., Owen, S., Pictor, S. P., & Paroski, M. W. (1991). Acquired cervical spine impairment in young adults with cerebral palsy. *Developmental Medicine and Child Neurology, 33,* 153–166.

Rosenbaum, D. (1991). *Human motor control.* San Diego: Academic Press.

Rosenthal, R. K. (1984). The use of orthotics in foot and ankle problems in cerebral palsy. *Foot and Ankle, 4*(4), 195–200.

Rutherford, M. A., Pennock, J. M., Murdoch-Eaton, D. M., Cowan, F. M., & Dubowitz, L. M. S. (1992). Athetoid cerebral palsy with cysts in the putamen after hypoxic-ischaemic encephalopathy. *Archives of Disease in Childhood, 67,* 846–850.

Sahrmann, S. (Ed.). (1983). Should there be NDT certification? View 1. *Physical Therapy, 63*(4), 552.

Sahrmann, S. A., & Norton, B. J. (1977). The relationship of voluntary movement to spasticity in the upper motor neuron syndrome. *Annals of Neurology, 2*(6), 460–465.

Schleichkorn, J. (1992). *The Bobaths: A biography of Berta and Karel Bobath.* Tucson, AZ: Therapy Skill Builders.

Schleichkorn, J. (1987). *"The Sometime Physician" William John Little: Pioneer in Treatment of Cerebral Palsy and Orthopedic Surgery.* Farmingdale, NY: Author

Schmahmann, J. D. (1991). An emerging concept: The cerebellar contribution to higher function. *Archives of Neurology, 48,* 1178–1187.

Scrutton, D. (Ed.). (1991). The Bobaths. *Developmental Medicine and Child Neurology, 33,* 565–566.

Shea, A. M. (1990). Growth and development in Down syndrome in infancy and early childhood: Implications for the physical therapist. In *Topics in Pediatrics: Lesson 5,* Alexandria, VA: American Physical Therapy Association.

Shumway-Cook, A., & Woollacott, M. H. (1985). Dynamics of postural control in the child with Down syndrome. *Physical Therapy, 65*(9), 1315–1322.

Shumway-Cook, A., & Woollacott, M. H. (1995). *Motor control: Theory and practical applications.* Baltimore, MD: Williams and Wilkins.

Simon, S. R., Deutsch, S. D., Nuzzo, R. M., Mansour, M. J., Jackson, J. L., Koskinen, M., & Rosenthal, R. K. (1978). Genu recurvatum in spastic cerebral palsy. *The Journal of Bone and Joint Surgery, 60-A*(7), 882–894.

Staheli, L. T. (1992). *Fundamentals of pediatric orthopedics.* New York: Raven Press.

Stallings, V. A., Charney, E. B., Davies, J. C., & Cronk, C. E. (1993a). Nutrition-related growth failure of children with quadriplegic cerebral palsy. *Developmental Medicine and Child Neurology, 35,* 126–138.

Stallings, V. A., Charney, E. B., Davies, J. C., & Cronk, C. E. (1993b). Nutritional status and growth of children with diplegic or hemiplegic cerebral palsy. *Developmental Medicine and Child Neurology, 35,* 997–1006.

Stamer, M. H. (1995). *Functional documentation: A process for the physical therapist.* San Antonio, TX: Therapy Skill Builders.

Stedman's Medical Dictionary (26th ed.). (1995). Baltimore: Williams and Wilkins.

Stevenson, R. D., Hayes, R. P., Cater, L. V., & Blackman J. A. (1994). Clinical correlates of linear growth in children with cerebral palsy. *Developmental Medicine and Child Neurology, 36,* 135–142.

Stevenson, R. D., Roberts, C. D., & Vogtle, L. (1995). The effects of non-nutritional factors on growth in cerebral palsy. *Developmental Medicine and Child Neurology, 37,* 124–130.

Styer-Acevedo, J. (1994). Physical therapy for the child with cerebral palsy. In J. Tecklin (Ed.), *Pediatric Physical Therapy* (pp. 89–130). Philadelphia: W. B. Saunders Co.

Sugden, D., & Utley, A. (1995). Interlimb coupling in children with hemiplegic cerebral palsy. *Developmental Medicine and Child Neurology, 37,* 293–309.

Sutherland, D. H. (1984). *Gait disorders in childhood and adolescence.* 128–151. Baltimore: Williams and Wilkins.

Sutherland, D. H., & Cooper, L. (1978). The pathomechanics of progressive crouch gait in spastic diplegia. *Orthopedic Clinics of North America, 9*(1), 143–154.

Tardieu, C., de la Tour, E. H., Bret, M. D., & Tardieu, G. (1982). Muscle hypoextensibility in children with cerebral palsy: I. Clinical and experimental observations. *Archives of Physical Medicine and Rehabilitation, 63,* 97–102.

Tardieu, C., Lesparot, A., Tabary, V., & Bret, M. D. (1988). For how long must the soleus muscle be stretched each day to prevent contracture? *Developmental Medicine and Child Neurology, 30,* 3–10.

Tardieu, G., Tardieu, C., Colbeau-Justin, P., & Lespargot, A. (1982). Muscle hypoextensibility in children with cerebral palsy: II. Therapeutic implications. *Archives of Physical Medicine and Rehabilitation, 63,* 103–107.

Thelen, E., Fisher, D. M., Ridley-Johnson, R., & Griffin, N. J. (1982). Effects of body build and arousal on newborn infant stepping. *Developmental Psychobiology, 25,* 447–453.

Thometz, J. G., & Simon, S. R. (1988). Progression of scoliosis after skeletal maturity in institutionalized adults who have cerebral palsy. *The Journal of Bone and Joint Surgery, 70-A*(9), 1290–1296.

Thorstensson, A., Carlson, H., Zomlefer, M. R., & Nilsson, J. (1982). Lumbar back muscle activity in relation to trunk movements during locomotion in man. *Acta Physiologica Scandinavica, 116,* 13–20.

U.S. Department of Health and Human Services. National Institutes of Health. (1993). *Research plan for the national center for medical rehabilitation research.* (NIH Publication No. 93-3509). Bethesda, MD: Author

Van den Berg-Emons, R. J. G., van Baak, M. A., de Barbanson, D. C., Speth, L., & Saris, W. H. M. (1996). Reliability of tests to determine peak aerobic power, anaerobic power and isokinetic muscle strength in children with spastic cerebral palsy. *Developmental Medicine and Child Neurology, 38,* 1117–1125.

Van der Meche, F. G. A., & Van Gijn, J. (1986). Hypotonia: An erroneous clinical concept? *Brain, 109,* 1169–1178.

Van Sant, A.(Ed.). (1983). Should there be NDT certification? View 5. *Physical Therapy, 63*(4), 554.

Walsh, E. G. (1992). *Muscles, masses, and motion. The physiology of normality, hypotonicity, spasticity and rigidity.* (Clinics in Developmental Medicine, Nos. 103, 125). New York: Cambridge University Press.

Wiklund, L. M., & Uvebrant, P. (1991). Hemiplegic cerebral palsy: Correlation between CT morphology and clinical findings. *Developmental Medicine and Child Neurology, 33,* 512–523.

Williams, P. E., & Goldspink, G. (1978). Changes in sarcomere length and physiological properties in immobilized muscle. *Journal of Anatomy, 127*(3), 459–468.

Yokochi, K., Shimabukuro, S., Kodama, M., Kodama, K., & Hosoe, A. (1993). Motor function of infants with athetoid cerebral palsy. *Developmental Medicine and Child Neurology, 35,* 909–916.

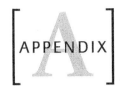

A Brief Summary of Normal Development

This summary of normal development gives the reader information against which to compare children with cerebral palsy. Although brief, the information presented can be used as a general guide in understanding some of the ways children developing without cerebral palsy learn their skills. It is based on clinical observations and on books by Bly (1994) and Alexander, Boehme, and Cupps (1993). Their books offer detailed information about normal development. Again, like the hypotheses that therapists make about children with CP, the conclusions that we draw about children developing normally have for the most part not been sufficiently researched.

Head, Neck, Tongue, Eyes

A child must learn control of the head and neck for the vital functions of ease of breathing, eating, speaking, and using the eyes to explore the environment. An infant is unable to control the head posturally for these functions and so must be ease of breathing, eating, speaking, and using the eyes to explore the environment. Infants first learn antigravity extension when held at their caregiver's shoulder or when placed in the prone position. Lifting the head is difficult because the head is proportionally large and the infant's trunk and hips flex, pushing the weight onto the head, especially in prone. Therefore the infant must work hard and tends to lift the head through small ranges at first from the surface it rests on. This hard work may be why the infant gains extension posturing and control slowly and smoothly throughout the cervical spine.

The structure of the infant's head, oral cavity, and ribcage give support for the feeding process so control of this area of the body need not be well-developed neurologically to successfully suck for nourishment. However, as the child extends the cervical area, jaw and tongue alignment are affected and begin to move separately from head movements. Active jaw, lip, and tongue movements develop with the feeding process as the head also is works to actively extend at the cervical spine. Control of the head on the neck and the neck on the thoracic spine depends on control of extension and flexion (especially the deep neck flexors and extensors). We think that the flexors and extensors work in a graded manner, creating a relationship of the muscles as they work together to control the head.

The ability to control the neck in the midranges of flexion and extension positioning seems critical in the ability to rotate the head. This is done first with support to the head in supine and then with support of the trunk and arms in prone. Moving the head in flexion, extension, and rotation enables the eyes to scan the environment. Because the neuromuscular system gives the child the options of these movements, the ability to initiate, sustain, or terminate them, and the ability to use them in different combinations (a variety of synergies), the child has options for placement of the eyes.

In addition, the biomechanical changes that take place during active, normal movement give the child options as to where the eyes can be placed. The extension of the spine as a whole, the descent of the ribcage, and the position assumed by the arms for support of various postures and transitional movements between postures gives the head and neck the support needed for movement in all three planes. Head control in all postures and transitional movements, therefore, depends on control of the trunk as a whole.

The effects of gravity also can assist head control or make it more difficult. Head control is easiest to first learn in supported, erect positions; that is, supported upright when an infant, or in sitting and standing. Prone is actually a very hard place to control the head, because of gravity and biomechanical considerations.

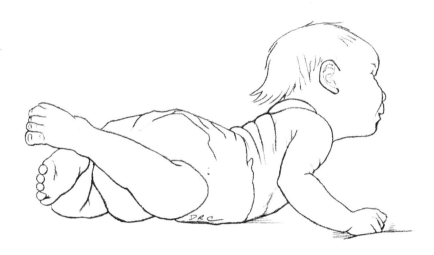

Figure 1   This 2-month-old baby uses extension of her head and upper trunk from an asymetrical starting position. She can push into the floor with her fists but must lift against gravity with this extension while working against the resistance of spinal and hip flexion. She uses upward gaze (eye extension) to assist the spinal extension.

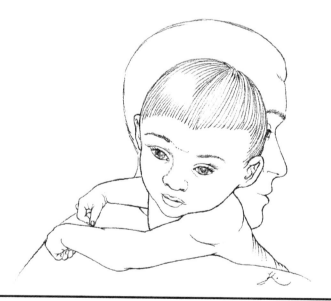

Figure 2   This 2-month-old is being held and carried on his father's shoulder. His trunk is well supported by his father's hands. Here, the baby does not have to contend with gravity as much as the baby in Figure 1 does, in order to lift his head. His position, supported by his father, also places the baby's trunk and hips in more extension, thereby making head lifting an easier task to learn.

The eyes play a significant role in postural control. Research has shown this even in very young infants (Butterworth & Hicks, 1977; Lee & Aronson, 1974; Shumway-Cook & Woollacott, 1995). Infants rely on visual cues to help sustain and guide head position and to balance. This is true in conflicting sensory environments experimentally, such as when the child's vision tells him he is moving, but his proprioceptive system tells him he is not. When infants who do not yet sit alone are placed in supported seats and the seat is not moving, but the walls around the infant move, the infant makes compensatory head movements as if he is losing balance.

Thoracic Spine, Ribcage, Upper Extremities

The thoracic spine and ribcage are rigid structures in the newborn that must become more mobile to allow for weight shift through the trunk and for graded respiration. There seems to be a strong relationship between the ability of the upper extremities to actively push into the surface they rest on and the ability to develop thoracic extension and descent of the ribcage. The infant uses the arms in prone and when supported upright against a caregiver to help lift the head by pushing down against the surface. This is probably done with pectoral and rotator cuff activity. The shoulder complex is elevated in an infant with the shoulders in extension and internal rotation. However, as the head and chest lift when the arms push, it becomes easier for the arms to move forward. The arms can then push with less elevation and more shoulder flexion and horizontal adduction. This changes the length-tension relationship of many of the muscles that attach to the clavicle, scapula, arm, and trunk. The likelihood of scapular stability, shoulder flexion and external rotation, and further thoracic extension increases as a result. This relationship also can be seen in any posture in which the trunk is well supported and the arms can push against a surface, such as sitting in a high chair. Moving the supported arms in front of the active trunk enables a more narrow base of push with the arms. The opportunity for weight shift from one arm to the other via active trunk movement of the flexors and extensors increases. This weight shift enables development of trunk movement in all three planes and for further strengthening of the arms. As the child gains control of the lower body for more upright posture, the upper trunk has been well prepared to support antigravity postures. The child uses the trunk for postural control and the arms for support as needed. Finally, the trunk is able to sustain nearly all postural needs to enable the arms the freedom of movement needed for reach, grasp, and manipulation.

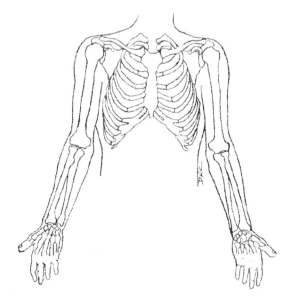

Figure 3 Skeletal anatomy of the adult's ribcage and upper extremities. Note the downward angle of the ribs and the nearly horizontal position of the clavicles.

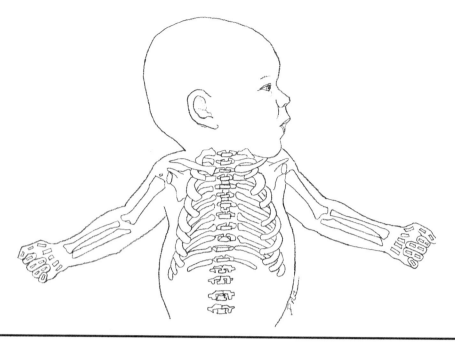

Figure 4   Skeletal anatomy of the infant's ribcage. Much of the skeleton is still cartilaginous. Note the more horizontal position of the ribs. The shape of the infant's ribcage has not been influenced yet by the pull of muscles and the shoulder complex is elevated.

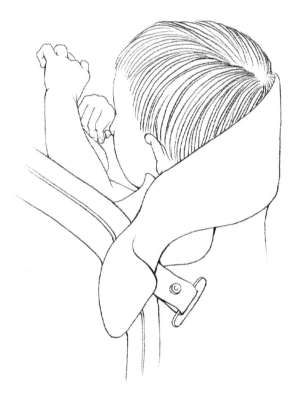

Figure 5a   This 2-month-old pushes into his mother's chest as he is carried facing her in a front pack carrier. This is a common way that infants under 3 months old practice pushing against a surface with their upper extremities.

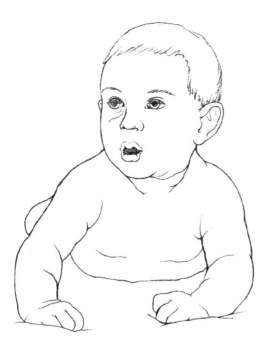

Figure 5b This 4-month-old pushes against the floor while in the prone position. He has less shoulder complex elevation now than the 2-month-old and is moving toward shoulder flexion. His shoulders are still quite internally rotated. He can shift weight onto the left arm, right his head so that his eyes remain horizontal, and rotate his head with control of cervical flexion and extension.

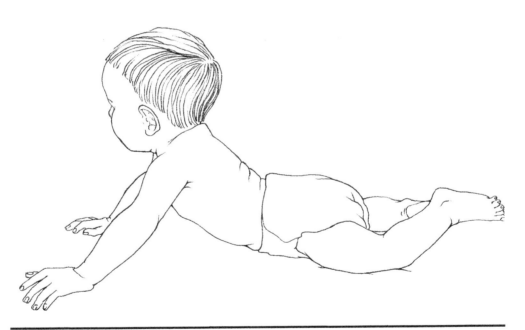

Figure 5c This 6-month-old shows the ability to extend her elbows when she pushes up in prone. An important point to this figure is that the baby not only uses thoracolumbar extension and elbow extension to lift herself up, but she also lifts the base of her ribcage up off of the floor with her abdominal muscles. This cocontraction of her lower trunk gives her the alignment to shift weight back onto her pelvis and legs and then to isometrically contract her hip extensors.

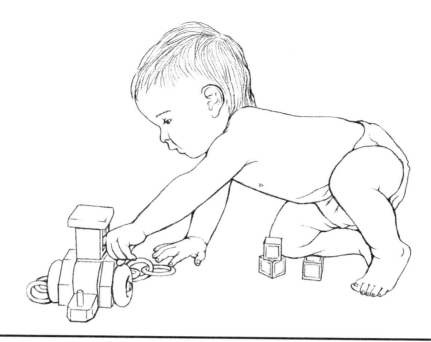

Figure 6 This 10-month-old controls his trunk in all three planes. Here he reaches while assuming, then sustaining, trunk extension with rotation. This rotation is a prerequisite for limb disassociation. Note also that this child is in a position that puts the latissimus dorsi muscle on the left in its most lengthened position.

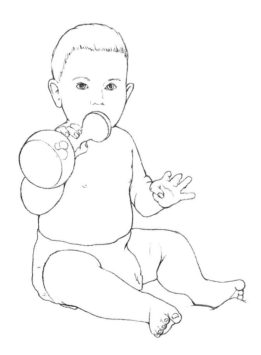

Figure 7 This 8-month-old can sit with arms free to play. He has developed control of his trunk extension and flexion as well as hip flexion and extension control. He assumes a wide base of support in this sitting position, which is a new skill for him. His wide base of support is a temporary musculoskeletal strategy that provides stability to trunk control in this new, upright position.

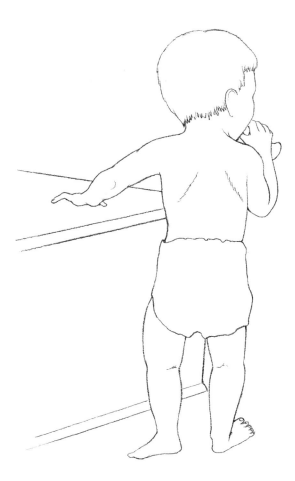

Figure 8 This 9-month-old is able to stand with support of one arm on a coffee table. This support widens her base of support and serves as a well-controlled pivot point to rotate to look as her father enters the room. She is able to rotate at the shoulder and hip joints as well as within the thoracic and cervical spine.

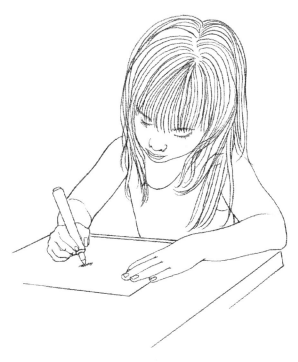

Figure 9 This 4-year-old holds her paper with her left hand as she writes. The subtle movement of her head and trunk in all three planes of movement helps her actively disassociate her arm movements to enable one arm to take weight while the other hand writes.

Thoracic Spine, Ribcage, Upper Extremities

The Lower Trunk

Because it houses the center of mass, the lower trunk is a critical area of the body for physical, occupational, and speech therapists to understand. The job of the lower trunk is to control the ribcage on the pelvis via muscular attachments. Muscular control is necessary for holding this area relatively still as the rest of the body moves, preventing the center of mass from moving excessively, and thus conserving energy. One of the main features of functional movement is that it is energy efficient.

The muscles that are primarily responsible for control of the lower trunk are the abdominal muscles, including the obliques, transverse abdominus, and rectus abdominus; and the trunk extensors which include the erector spinae, deeper extensors (multifidus and rotators), quadratus lumborum, and latissimus dorsi. Posteriorly there are more superficial muscles that assist respiration, (such as the serratus posterior), that can be included in the list of muscles necessary to control the lower trunk.

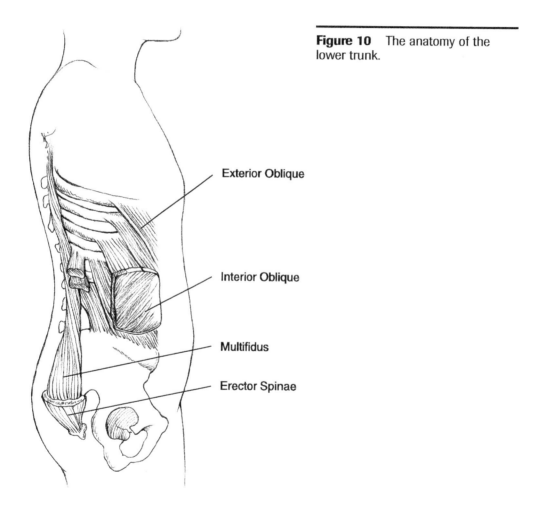

Figure 10 The anatomy of the lower trunk.

Exterior Oblique

Interior Oblique

Multifidus

Erector Spinae

During normal development, the infant must change the lumbar curve from the initial position of flexion to lumbar extension or lordosis. This is done first mechanically, as the infant works to push against a surface with the upper body in prone or supported upright with contact to the ventral surface of the body. It also can be seen in bridging activities in supine or arching when rolling. The lumbar curve slowly develops as the upper trunk and upper extremities are active in their antigravity work. The curve develops later in sitting, standing, and on all fours. It becomes active as the infant pushes up higher with upper extremities against a surface or extends the entire spine to move, as in rolling. Because the hip flexors are not fully lengthened in an infant and influence the position of the lumbar spine via their attachments to the lumbar vertebrae, extension of the lumbar spine pulls against these tight hip flexors. The result is a pronounced lumbar lordosis while the hip flexors gradually lengthen to allow full hip extension.

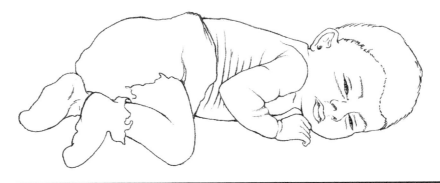

Figure 11a   The newborn shows lumbar flexion in all positions she is placed or held.

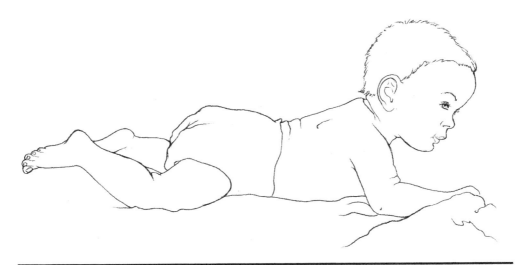

Figure 11b   At 3 months, this baby uses active cervical and upper thoracic extension to lift his head. His arms also push into the support surface. He is beginning to gain range of lumbar extension because of the activity and alignment of the upper body and because of the end range tightness of his hip flexors pulling on the lumbar spine as his pelvis takes his body weight against the floor.

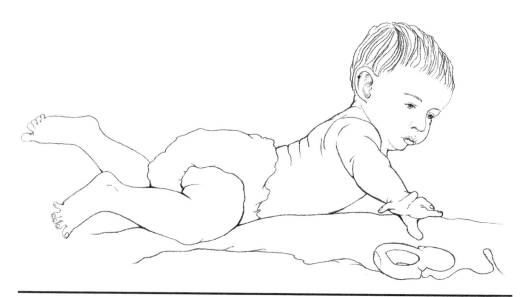

Figure 11c At 6 months, this baby uses active trunk extension through the lumbar spine and is beginning to use holding with the hip extensors while the anterior part of the pelvis is flat against the support surface.

At the same time, the infant is practicing movements that require the use of the abdominal muscles. The abdominal muscles are the flexors of the lower trunk and stabilize the ribcage onto the pelvis. In supine, the infant often first lifts the lower extremities with the hip flexors only, but as he lifts them higher, and the buttocks lift from the surface, the abdominal muscles assist the movement. The abdominal muscles also are active in any trunk rotation activity, which is normally seen beginning in the second half of the first year. Rotation with extension of the spine is seen in prone, sitting, sit to all fours and back, and standing supported. Rotation with flexion of the lower trunk is seen in supine play, rolling supine to prone, and lifting the legs while sitting on the floor. Rotation is a complex synergy requiring control and interaction of both flexors and extensors of the trunk. This is why it is so often missing in children with cerebral palsy. Rotation is a desired movement in many functions because it tends to keep the lower trunk, which is the center of mass, in a relatively steady position. Any movement that enables the child a skilled function yet does not cause the center of mass to move much conserves energy.

The child also uses the abdominal muscles toward the end of the first year to grade and prolong exhalation for vocalization. Remember that the abdominal muscles stabilize the ribcage distally to the pelvis. This helps change the shape of the ribcage from its infant elevation and horizontal rib structure to a more downward-angled, less elevated position. The abdominal muscles are responsible for holding the abdominal contents in place, and for resisting the diaphragm on inspiration so that excessive movement of the belly does not occur. Along with the intercostals, which anatomically are part of the abdominal obliques, the abdominal muscles assist controlled exhalation by grading muscle activity.

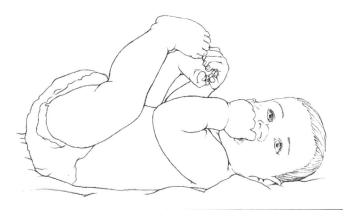

Figure 12 At about 6 months, the baby can lift his legs toward his mouth. As movement is initiated from the legs and lower trunk, the abdominal muscles become more active in stabilizing the lower trunk. Note that this is accomplished with the trunk supported in extension. The more the pelvis lifts up from the support surface, the more the lower abdominal muscles are recruited.

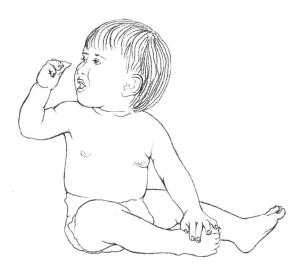

Figure 13a This 9-month-old is able to combine postural extensor and flexor muscles of the trunk to produce rotation. Rotation of the trunk enables the baby to look behind him. Rotation also enables smooth, graded transitions between postures while keeping the center of mass from moving excessively. In this movement to look behind him, the baby keeps the lower trunk in extension while rotating.

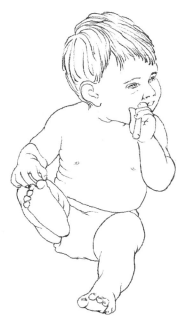

Figure 13b This baby also can keep his trunk in extension in the thoracic spine, then begin to move out of lumbar extension when using his abdominal muscles to assist lifting his legs. In this way, the baby shifts his weight toward the back of his base of support. Therapists often describe this posture as moving toward a posterior pelvic tilt. While this is true, the therapist must pay particular attention to what muscular activity throughout the trunk and lower extremities is producing this change in alignment of the pelvis.

The Lower Trunk

The Pelvic Girdle and Lower Extremities

The lower extremities serve as an active, stable base of support for movement elsewhere in the body and for controlled mobility from a stable trunk for movement. The lower extremities start out in development as a stable base of support. The hip joints are positioned in flexion, abduction, and external rotation in all early postures of the infant. This helps keep the base of support wide as the infant begins work with the upper body. It is with this wide base that the infant also initially learns active support in the lower extremities. This is seen in early prone, supine, and supported sitting postures as the trunk and upper body become more active in antigravity positions. Yet the lower extremities are not still or inactive even during these early postures; the legs kick in supine, push in prone, and begin to push down against the surface in sitting. The base of support in any posture does not narrow until the baby has control of the entire trunk in all three planes. This is an important relationship that therapists must remember during treatment.

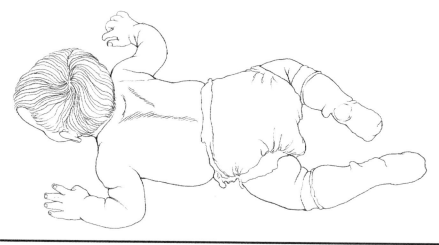

Figure 14a This 4-month-old is active in upper trunk extension. As the head lifts and weight is shifted toward the lower body, his hip flexion, abduction, and external rotation provide a wide base of support to assist in his newly achieved antigravity upper trunk extension.

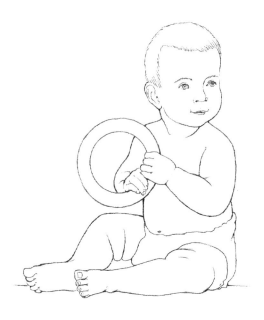

Figure 14b This 8-month-old is active in trunk extension through the entire spine and has some control of hip flexion and extension in sitting weight shifting. He maintains a wide base of support in sitting with hip flexion, abduction, and external rotation, which enables mechanical stability in a wide base of support. Because of this, he does not yet have to control lateral weight shifting or rotation in the trunk, nor does he have to control hip abduction/adduction to stay upright in sitting.

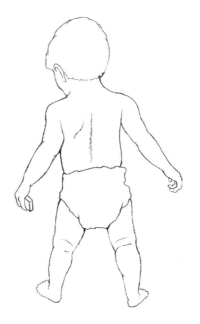

Figure 14c This 12-month-old reverts to a wide base of support by abducting his hips, which also are externally rotated, to assist with his new standing alone skill. He also uses shoulder extension with scapular adduction to assist trunk extension.

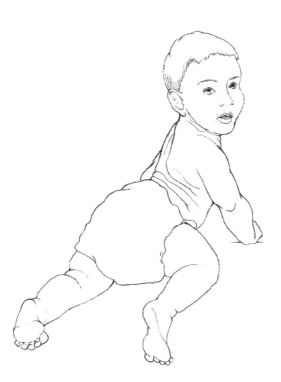

Figure 15a This 5-month-old actively rotates his trunk while supported on the floor to look behind him. Control of the entire trunk in all three planes assists active limb disassociation of the uppers and lowers. The weight-bearing left upper extremity is in more scapular adduction with less elevation than the right. The left lower extremity is in more hip extension and adduction with less external rotation than the right.

The Pelvic Girdle and Lower Extremities

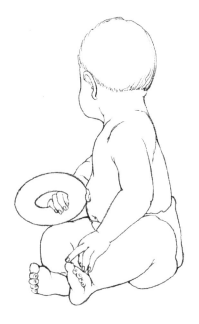

Figure 15b The 8-month-old seen in Figure 14b begins to narrow his base of support as he uses cervical and upper thoracic rotation to look and listen around him. By turning to the right, he shifts weight onto his right hip, which enables more lateral contact of the hip against the floor. The more he shifts onto this hip, the more the abductor on the right can actively assist sitting balance. If the baby were to rotate his trunk further to the right without losing control, his left hip would begin to adduct and internally rotate. In normal development, the hips do not move into a position of internal rotation until the trunk is controlled in all three planes.

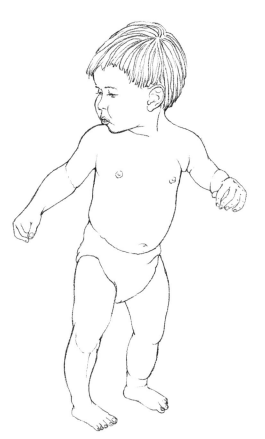

Figure 15c At 12 months, this baby is able to use trunk rotation and visually guided movement to look behind him. This begins to decrease the hip abduction and external rotation that the baby first stands alone with. Note how the activity of the baby's vision and trunk cause medial and lateral movements in his feet.

The second function of the pelvic girdle and lower extremities is controlled mobility. The legs are often the base of support for many positions and transitional movements (movements between postures or positions). Yet they also must move themselves, as in moving from sitting to standing, from all fours to sitting, and in walking. They must be able to work alternately as an active base of support and as mobile parts of the body that take the child somewhere. In development, this seems to be prepared for as the child alternately stabilizes with the lower extremities and moves the trunk, then stabilizes with the trunk and upper extremities and moves the lower extremities. Ultimately, the child is then able to move the trunk and lower extremities at the same time with the center of mass moving very little in order to conserve energy.

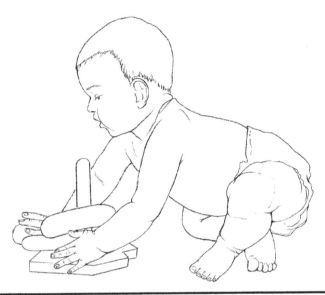

Figure 16 A 9- to 12-month-old often spends a good part of his playing time moving between all fours and sitting. Babies at this age will stop at any point during this transitional movement to reach, look, and listen. This 9-month-old can dis- associate lower extremity movement. This is possible because the trunk is actively posi- tioned in rotation. As he moves across a weight-bearing foot, he can concentrically and eccentrically contract different muscles around the hip, knee, and ankle joints, depending on the position of the leg and the direction of movement.

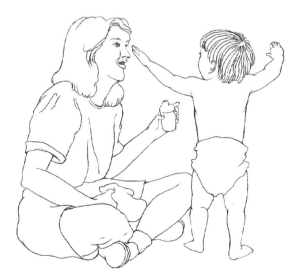

Figure 17 This 9-month-old can stand supported with one hand holding onto the window frame. He can reach toward his mother while keeping his trunk over the center of his base of support. His hips are abducted so that his feet are placed slightly wider than the width of his pelvis.

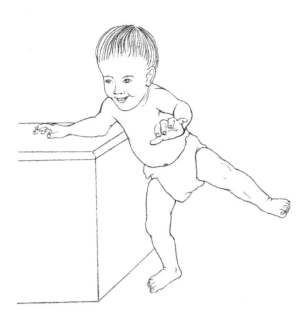

Figure 18 This 9-month-old girl momentarily lost her balance as she was walking with one arm supported on the coffee table. Here she shows an equilibrium reaction with the limbs on the unweighted side of her body abducting to regain the position of her center of mass over her base of support. It is possible for her to abduct these limbs, however, only because the weight bearing limbs actively push into the support surfaces of the coffee table and floor with isometric contractions of muscle groups that stabilize the weight bearing joints.

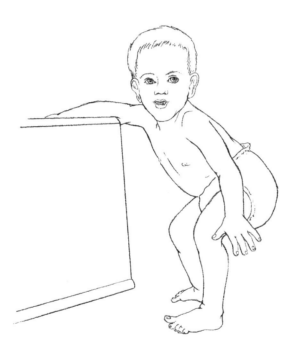

Figure 19 This 10-month-old is able to begin squatting to retrieve toys on the floor or to control a stand to floor transition. With her arm on the coffee table widening her base of support and actively pushing down on the table, she begins to grade eccentric extension of the hip, knee, and ankle.

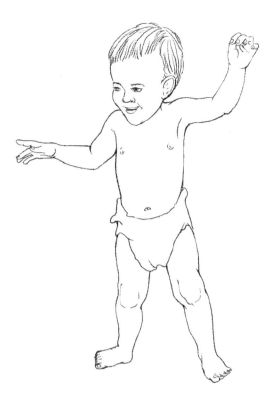

Figure 20 This 11-month-old is standing alone for the first time. Her arms move into shoulder abduction and external rotation and her scapulae adduct to assist thoracic extension to stay upright. She widens her base of support in her lower body to achieve this new skill as she is no longer widening it with an arm on a support surface.

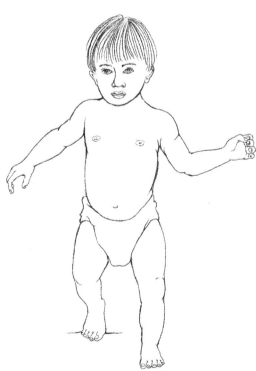

Figure 21 This 12-month-old is taking independent steps. The new skill is performed with shoulders in slight elevation and external rotation to assist active thoracic extension. His hips are abducted and externally rotated, maintaining slight hip flexion throughout the stance and swing portions of each step.

The Pelvic Girdle and Lower Extremities

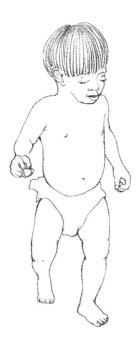

Figure 22   At 17 months, this same child incorporates trunk rotation into his walking, which enables a longer step length. His hips also are less abducted and externally rotated.

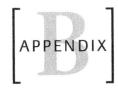

Cocontraction

Cocontraction is the "simultaneous activity of agonist and antagonist muscles crossing the same joint and acting in the same plane" (Damiano, 1993). It is controlled by the neuromuscular system and allows for increased stiffness of the joint. *Stiffness* is a dynamic relationship of the joint's angular movement and resistance of that joint to the angular forces. Forces may be extrinsic, such as gravity or a weight placed on the limb, or intrinsic, such as soft tissue extensibility and muscle activity. The central nervous system has a role in changing joint stiffness by influencing muscle activity around the joint. Usually, the more the muscles around the joint contract, the stiffer the joint becomes. But cocontraction and the opposite end of the continuum, reciprocal inhibition (the contraction of the agonist with the simultaneous inhibition of the antagonist), do not usually occur in their strict definitions in skilled posture and movement control. Rather, the neuromuscular system grades or scales the relationship of agonist and antagonist activity around the joint to meet the demand of the function. This becomes more and more refined in its timing and sequencing of muscle activity the more skilled one becomes.

Cocontraction is one way that the central nervous system can increase stiffness of the limb or joint in order to limit degrees of freedom at that joint; that is, limit the number of planes a joint or limb has to control. It is an effective and desirable way to stabilize the joint that may require less complex neural functions than graded agonist/antagonist activity during joint movement. In young children developing normally, cocontraction serves the purpose of stabilizing joints against unexpected forces or against lack of more complex movements that would require graded muscle activity that the child does not yet have. We attribute this ability of the young child to first use cocontraction as a function of a maturing neurological system that develops spinal and supraspinal inhibition over time.

What is most interesting, however, is that older children and adults who are learning a new skill also tend to use cocontraction with muscle activity in distant joints (unnecessary overactivity). With practice of the new skill (motor learning), coordination, which is the timing and ordering of muscle activation patterns, changes, so that appropriate graded activity and energy efficiency specific to the skill emerge. Cocontraction also can increase at certain joints if this is necessary for the skill.

Children with spasticity (positive sign) often use too much cocontraction with loss of graded agonist/antagonist relationships (negative sign) in gait (Berger, et al., 1982; Leonard, et al., 1991). On the other hand, children with Down syndrome have difficulty using cocontraction with sufficient intensity and duration, which appears to affect their motor function (Davis and Kelso, 1982).

As a pediatric therapist practicing in the clinic, you may have observed that children with hypotonia often cannot generate sufficient cocontraction for functional skills. Since cocontraction seems to be one of the initial ways the neuromuscular system generates postural stability, this may be where treatment should begin. On the other hand, a child with hypertonia who uses excessive cocontraction has generated some patterns of antigravity postural control. In this case, your job will be to decrease excessive and non-functional cocontraction while ensuring sufficient and functional cocontraction to perform skills.

You also can use the knowledge of the recruitment of cocontraction or excessive activity of muscles when assisting children in learning new skills. For example, when teaching a child to stand alone for the first time, try to achieve alignment that allows maximal use of trunk extension with hip extension. Extension often is learned and used first in new skills. Help limit the degrees of freedom at the lumbar spine and hip by placing the hip in about 10–15 degrees of flexion (to assist a very slight anterior pelvic tilt which facilitates lumbar extension) and external rotation. This limits the joint movement that the child has to control in the trunk by placing the lumbar facet joints in extension (the close packed position). The external rotation of the hips increases the base of support and facilitates the best length-tension relationship for the gluteus maximus to extend the hip. Then support the child at the lower trunk and/or hips and tilt him forward slightly so that the postural reaction needs to be one of extension, but with slight flexion at the hips so that active flexion may cocontract with the extensors. The knee and ankle extensors also are recruited with this alignment and postural reaction.

You may tell children and their parents that when children try new skills they can expect that their bodies will work harder. The child with mild to moderately hypotonicity often tries and sometimes achieves postural stiffness that for a while may interfere with graded control, but yet enables him to begin to practice antigravity control. The child with hypertonicity often uses his excessive cocontraction to attempt the new skill. Tell them to expect this, not to be too worried that they are doing this, and that you will work through it.

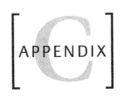

APPENDIX

Examples of superficial muscles, two-joint muscles, and muscles that were originally shortened at birth.

Superficial muscles

cervical erector spinae

pectoralis major

biceps brachii

hamstrings

long toe flexors

scapular elevators

latissimus dorsi

long finger flexors

gastrocnemious

Two (or more) joint muscles

latissimus dorsi

rectus femoris

psoas major

long finger flexors

gastrocnemious

biceps brachii (long head)

hamstrings

gracilis

long toe flexors

Muscles that are short at birth

suprahyoid muscles

pectorals

intercostals

quadratus lumborum

long finger flexors

thenar muscles

hamstrings

long toe flexors

scapular elevators

latissimus dorsi

rectus abdominus

biceps brachii

forearm pronators

hip flexors

rectus femoris

INDEX

A

activities of daily living (ADLs), 7, 39
  eating, 7
alignment, 5, 11, 27, 33, 37, 45–47, 52, 54, 58, 60, 65–69, 78–79, 81, 83, 85, 87–89, 91–92, 94, 98, 101, 105–108, 114, 116–117, 121–122, 132–133, 136, 139, 142–143, 150–151, 173–174, 177, 179, 181, 186, 203, 207, 227, 231, 235, 237, 246
alignment,
  abnormal, 78, 105, 114
  normal, 83, 150–151
ankle, 52–53, 68–69, 71, 77, 105, 115–116, 130, 133, 143, 147–148, 204, 212, 241–242, 246
ankle,
  in children with athetosis, 143, 147
  in children with hypertonia, 77, 143
arousal/attention, 16–17, 47, 67
ataxia, 9–10, 13–14, 67, 115, 189–207, 209, 211–213, 215, 217
  classifications of, 189
athetoid, 9, 18, 21, 28, 141, 143–144, 165
athetosis, 9–10, 13, 28, 48, 67, 72, 80, 101, 141–187, 191, 194, 196, 204, 211
  classifications of, 141
auditory processing, 194, 200

B

balance, 72, 82, 86, 90, 113, 115, 144, 170, 182, 184, 202, 204, 229, 240, 242
basal ganglia, 141, 143
base of support, 24–25, 29, 39, 42–47, 49–52, 55, 57, 60–61, 68–69, 83, 86–91, 94–95, 98–99, 102–103, 105, 108, 113–116, 118–123, 149, 163, 165–168, 170–171, 198, 202–206, 208, 211–213, 217, 232–233, 237–243, 246
biomechanics, 45, 74, 77, 112, 130
Bobath, 3–5, 9, 14, 64, 67

C

cardiorespiratory endurance, 16–17
center of mass, 24, 27, 41–42, 44, 55, 67–69, 82–83, 86–87, 90–91, 98–99, 103, 105, 109–110, 112–113, 115, 119, 122, 130, 149, 161, 165, 177, 192, 195, 202–205, 234, 236–237, 241–242
cerebellum (cerebellar), 21, 141, 189–195, 200, 211
cerebral palsy, 1, 3–7, 9–22, 24, 29, 34, 41, 63–64, 68–70, 73–74, 76, 97, 141, 143–144, 149, 157, 165, 189–195, 201, 211–212, 227, 236
cervical, 28, 32–33, 37, 43, 57–58, 79, 104–106, 108, 155, 167, 174, 208, 233, 240, 247
  extension, 18, 25, 27, 31–33, 35–37, 39–41, 46, 50, 55, 60, 79–83, 86, 101–102, 108,

111, 113, 125–127, 145, 147–151, 153, 156, 160–162, 164, 166–167, 170–171, 174, 177, 180–182, 185, 198, 202, 227, 231, 235
  flexion, 31, 37, 45, 78, 81, 83, 150–151, 153, 155, 208, 231
  rotation, 18, 43, 83, 126, 174, 233, 240
  spine, 18, 25, 27, 31, 33, 36, 40, 45, 47, 78–82, 86, 104–106, 108, 126–127, 147–151, 153, 156, 160–161, 167, 174, 185, 198, 202, 208, 227, 233
chorea, 142
choreoathetosis, 142, 194
cocontraction, 5, 10, 12–13, 18, 21–23, 40–41, 45, 48, 64–67, 71, 77, 90, 93, 101, 106, 131, 144, 165, 181, 192, 195, 199, 203–204, 206, 231, 245–246
  compensatory, 67
  excessive, 63, 66–67, 71, 96, 113, 142, 195, 206, 245–246
  normal, 192
  sustained, 22, 63–67, 77, 106, 115, 130
communication, 6, 39, 81, 101, 144, 151, 155, 164, 196

D

deep tendon reflexes (DTR), 12, 22, 143, 191
degrees of freedom, 245–246
depth perception, 33, 69, 81, 122, 124
digestion, 17, 36
diplegia, 9, 63–64, 66, 78, 104–125, 128, 164, 168, 191–192, 195, 205–206
disabilities, 1, 3–4, 6–7, 9, 16, 18–20, 33, 39, 41–42, 44, 64, 81, 84, 87, 90, 106, 109, 113, 116, 126, 128, 130, 132, 142, 144, 150, 152, 155, 160, 162, 165–166, 170–171, 189, 192, 198, 200, 203, 206, 211–212
dislocation,
  hip, 28–29, 74–76, 88, 114, 148, 164, 167
  shoulder, 28–29, 147
Down syndrome, 10–11, 21, 24, 29, 245
dyskinesia, 142
dysmetria, 189–190, 196
dystonia, 142

E

elbow, 23–24, 34, 38, 40, 60–61, 83–84, 93, 96, 99, 107, 109, 127, 139, 192, 200, 203, 231
  in children with athetosis, 144, 148–149, 155–157, 161–162, 171–172, 182–184, 222
  in children with hypertonia, 65, 157
  in children with hypotonia, 29
  in normal development, 144

N

National Center for Medical Rehabilitation Research (NCMRR), 6–7, 10–11, 18
negative signs of central nervous system dysfunction, 10–11, 21, 63–64, 245
Neurodevelopmental Treatment (NDT), 4–6, 9–10, 65, 94
neuromuscular synergies, 12, 116
   in children with ataxia, 199
   in children with hypertonia, 67–68, 71
neuromuscular system, 6, 11–13, 15, 17, 22–25, 41, 64–68, 143–144, 156, 191–192, 227, 245
normal development, 5–6, 11–12, 15–17, 35, 42, 60, 75, 79, 83, 106, 125, 192, 196, 199, 212, 227–244
nutrition, 14, 16–17, 20, 33, 71, 78, 81, 151, 155

O

ordering of muscle firing, 67
oscillations, 21, 93

P

pathophysiology, 6–7, 10–11, 16, 21, 24, 63–64, 88, 141–143, 152, 189–191
periventricular white matter, 64
positive signs of central nervous system dysfunction, 10, 21, 63–64, 196, 245
postural control, 5, 13, 15–17, 19, 21, 25, 34–36, 41, 45, 47, 49–50, 57–59, 66–67, 79, 82, 90–92, 94, 101, 105, 117, 144, 147, 153, 165–166, 171–172, 193, 195–198, 203–204, 206, 212, 227–229, 238, 245–246
postural muscles, 12, 15–17, 24–26, 28–29, 40–42, 47–48, 54, 59–60, 67, 72–73, 79, 85–87, 91, 102, 153, 195, 237
primary impairments, 11, 13–14, 16–17
   in children with ataxia, 193
   in children with athetosis, 144–145, 171
   in children with hypertonia, 66, 68–71, 73, 77–79, 81, 104, 116, 126
   in children with hypotonia, 22, 24–26, 29, 33–34, 40–41, 59
proprioception, 5, 239
   in children with ataxia, 14, 189–191, 194, 207, 222
   in children with athetosis, 13, 146–147, 194
   in children with hypertonia, 13, 69–70, 125
   in children with hypotonia, 13, 25, 33, 46–47, 193–194
   in normal development, 13

Q

quadriplegia, 9, 63–64, 66, 72–73, 79–103, 108, 114, 125, 148

R

reciprocal inhibition, 4, 10, 12, 65–66, 113, 192, 245
reflexive (reflexes), 4, 145
   primitive, 157
   tone, 5, 10, 12, 22, 63–64, 90, 143, 191
respiration, 229, 234
   in children with ataxia, 195–197, 200–203
   in children with athetosis, 151, 160, 162, 165, 180

   in children with hypertonia, 72, 78–79, 84, 87, 94, 97, 110, 112–113
   in children with hypotonia, 26, 29–30, 36–37, 39, 42, 46, 54, 59
ribcage, 15–16
   in children with ataxia, 195–196, 199–201, 203, 213
   in children with athetosis, 156, 158, 160, 162, 165, 180
   in children with hypertonia, 71–72, 74, 75, 78–79, 81–84, 86–87, 92–93, 95, 102–103–106, 108, 110, 111, 117, 123, 126, 127, 136
   in children with hypotonia, 26–27, 29–30, 34–36, 39, 46–49, 52, 54
   in normal development, 16, 30, 227, 229–231, 233–234, 236

S

scoliosis, 72–74, 86, 132, 149, 164–165, 167
secondary impairments, 3, 11, 13–15
   in children with ataxia, 193, 195–196, 199
   in children with athetosis, 145, 147–148, 151, 160
   in children with hypertonia, 65, 67–73, 77–78
   in children with hypotonia, 24–26, 28–29, 31, 33–34, 40–42, 45, 195
sensory feedback, 11, 13, 18, 31, 39, 70, 73, 138, 144, 193
sensory systems, 3–6, 11–13, 17, 26, 229
   in children with ataxia, 14, 189–190, 192–200, 203, 206, 209, 211–214
   in children with athetosis, 141, 144–147
   in children with hypertonia, 63, 68–71, 73, 81, 94, 104, 119, 124, 127–129, 131–132, 135–139
   in children with hypotonia, 25–26, 31, 39, 47
shoulder complex, 31–32, 35–37, 39, 57, 60, 72, 78, 82–84, 103, 106–108, 117, 127, 156–157, 161, 166, 182–183, 196, 199, 230–231
sitting, 19, 26, 31, 36, 39, 41–42, 44–45, 47, 49, 51, 60, 62, 69, 74, 82, 84–86, 90–91, 94, 99, 106, 108–109, 112–114, 116, 119, 122, 129, 148–149, 151, 155–156, 161, 165, 167–168. 171, 180, 182, 186, 198, 200–201, 203, 206–207, 212, 217, 228–229, 232, 235–236, 238, 240–241
skeletal deformities, 14, 40, 72, 86, 91, 114, 116, 147
skin conditions, 16–17, 26, 73, 165
societal limitations, 7, 9, 18–20, 39
spasticity, 4, 10, 18, 63–64, 67, 72, 80, 90, 101, 108, 143, 148, 166, 168, 176–177, 180–181, 192, 199, 206, 245
speech, 13, 16–17, 30, 42, 47, 52, 54, 57, 79, 81, 84, 101, 116, 120, 122, 126, 132, 136, 170, 172, 180–181, 195, 197, 199–200, 203, 210, 214, 234
spine, 16, 18, 25, 29, 31–37, 43, 45–48, 54, 58, 60, 62, 65–66, 72, 74–75, 78–83, 85–87, 90–91, 95, 98, 100, 104–113, 116, 118–119, 125–129, 134–135, 147–153, 156, 158, 160–165, 167–168, 170–171, 174, 179–180, 185, 202–203, 208–209, 212, 216, 227, 229–238, 246